Molecules from Side Reactions II

Molecules from Side Reactions II

Editors

Stefano D'Errico
Annalisa Guaragna

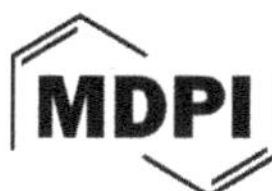

Basel • Beijing • Wuhan • Barcelona • Belgrade • Novi Sad • Cluj • Manchester

Editors

Stefano D'Errico
University of Naples
Federico II
Naples
Italy

Annalisa Guaragna
University of Naples
Federico II
Naples
Italy

Editorial Office
MDPI
St. Alban-Anlage 66
4052 Basel, Switzerland

This is a reprint of articles from the Special Issue published online in the open access journal *Molbank* (ISSN 1422-8599) (available at: https://www.mdpi.com/journal/molbank/special_issues/side_reaction_II).

For citation purposes, cite each article independently as indicated on the article page online and as indicated below:

Lastname, A.A.; Lastname, B.B. Article Title. *Journal Name* **Year**, *Volume Number*, Page Range.

ISBN 978-3-0365-9282-4 (Hbk)
ISBN 978-3-0365-9283-1 (PDF)
doi.org/10.3390/books978-3-0365-9283-1

Contents

About the Editors

Stefano D'Errico

Stefano D'Errico is an Assistant Professor in Organic Chemistry at the Department of Pharmacy of University of Naples Federico II. He finished his doctoral studies in 2009, with a thesis titled "Synthesis and structural characterization of quadruplex forming oligonucleotides and studies on solid phase synthesis of nucleoside and nucleotide analogues". His research activities focus mainly on the development of innovative synthetic methodologies for the preparation of novel bioactive modified nucleosides and nucleotides, and on the solid-phase synthesis of oligonucleotides to be exploited in the fields of medicinal and supramolecular chemistry. He has participated in several scientific projects, received two awards for the scientific research and is author of more than 70 papers published in international peer-reviewed journals.

Annalisa Guaragna

Annalisa Guaragna is an Associate Professor of Organic Chemistry at the Department of Chemical Science of the University of Naples Federico II. She obtained her MD in Biological Sciences in 1994 and a PhD in Chemical Sciences in 1999 from the University of Naples. Her scientific interests are mainly focused in the Bioorganic Chemistry area, particularly in the development of efficient synthetic methodologies and their application to the synthesis of diverse biologically relevant compounds, especially those for therapeutic applications in the field of infectious and rare diseases. She worked on the synthesis of glycomimetics, including natural, non-natural carbohydrates and iminosugars, on the synthesis of biomimetics such as sugar-modified nucleosides and nucleic acids analogues, and on the synthesis of new drug delivery systems. Much of Guaragna's research has been published in peer-reviewed papers in international journals, including 70 papers mainly as the first or corresponding author and 4 invited book chapters.

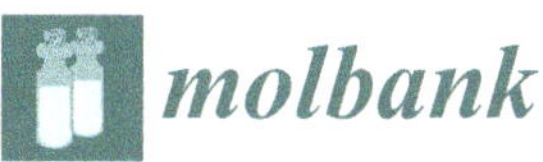 molbank MDPI

Editorial

Editorial: Special Issue "Molecules from Side Reactions II"

Stefano D'Errico [1,*] and Annalisa Guaragna [2]

[1] Department of Pharmacy, University of Naples Federico II, via Domenico Montesano 49, 80131 Naples, Italy
[2] Department of Chemical Sciences, University of Naples Federico II, via Cintia 21, 80126 Naples, Italy; guaragna@unina.it
* Correspondence: stefano.derrico@unina.it

This Special Issue, "Molecules from Side Reactions II", belongs to the section Organic Synthesis of the journal *Molbank* and was launched in 2021, after the first edition, "Molecules from Side Reactions". "Molecules from Side Reactions I&II" have collected brief papers dealing with the synthesis and characterization of molecules obtained from unexpected and/or unpredictable synthetic routes.

Research concerning side products deserves to be published for at least these two main reasons: (1) side products can be useful starting points and/or intermediates for new syntheses and (2) the rationalization of the reaction conditions through which they were formed might allow for a better understanding of reaction mechanisms.

It is pleasing to see that both Special Issues have been considered useful forums of discussion for research addressing side products by organic chemists of different nationalities.

Within two years, "Molecules from Side Reactions II" collected 17 papers, with Italy being the country that contributed the most research (Figure 1). The geographical attribution was derived from the affiliations of corresponding authors.

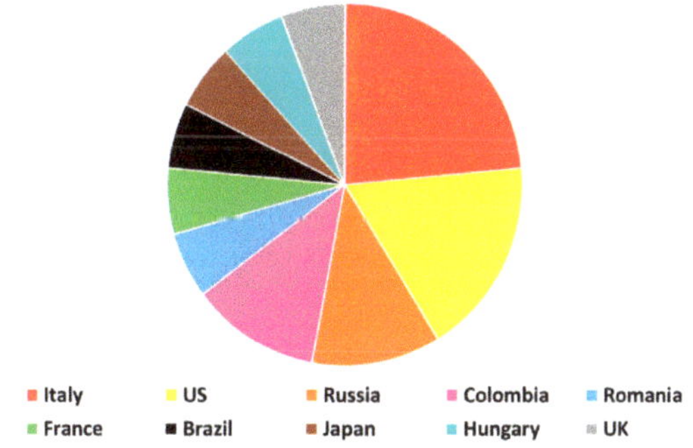

Figure 1. Geographical distribution of manuscripts belonging to the Special Issue "Molecules from Side Reactions II".

Citation: D'Errico, S.; Guaragna, A. Editorial: Special Issue "Molecules from Side Reactions II". *Molbank* **2023**, *2023*, M1740. https://doi.org/10.3390/M1740

Received: 17 October 2023
Accepted: 19 October 2023
Published: 20 October 2023

This Special Issue's topics cover the following aspects of organic chemistry:

- Synthesis of heterocycles;
- Synthesis of carbohydrates;
- Synthesis of modified nucleosides;
- Mechanisms of reactions;
- Green Chemistry;
- Chemistry of natural substances.

A summary of the research results published in this Special Issue follows.

Politano et al. found that the treatment of ethyl 2-oxocyclohexanecarboxylate with 4-acetamido-2,2,6,6-tetramethylpiperidine-1-oxoammonium tetrafluoroborate produced, unexpectedly, ethyl salicylate instead of ethyl 2-oxo-3-cyclohexene-1-carboxylate (contribution 1). The discovered methodology has the following advantages over conventional oxidative dehydrogenation reactions [1]: (1) the conversion is metal-free, and (2) the oxoammonium salt oxidant is environmentally friendly [2].

Tetrazoles are non-natural heterocyclic compounds endowed with interesting biological properties [3]. To obtain these compounds, Sepsey Für et al. studied the reaction of pyridazinethiones with hydrazine (contribution 2). Together with the expected *E* and *Z* stereoisomers of the desired hydrazones, they surprisingly recovered small amounts of the Schiff bases obtained after the reaction of the hydrazones with acetone present in traces in the glassware.

With the aim to decorate the bioactive isoindolo[2,1-*a*]quinoline scaffold [4], exploiting a Claisen–Schmidt-type condensation reaction [5], Rodríguez et al. obtained a new *N*-{2-[(3-oxo-1,3-dihydro-2-benzofuran-1-yl)acetyl]phenyl}acetamide derivative as a side-product (contribution 3).

Multivalent carbohydrates can recognize proteins on cell surfaces and induce biological effects [6,7]. Multivalency has been mimicked artificially by synthesizing polymers containing carbohydrates, functionalized with linkers at the end of which a polymerizable acrylamide moiety can be introduced [8]. When Miyagawa et al. studied the acryloylation reaction of 6-aminohexyl α-D-mannoside (contribution 4), they isolated both the desired *N*-hexyl α-D-acetylmannosyl acrylamide and the unknown *N*,*N*-bis(hexyl α-D-acetylmannosyl) acrylamide monomer, which contains two hexyl mannose units and one acrylamide group.

Rachid et al., noted the unexpected formation of an oxazole ring during the synthesis of a copper(I) cyanide network polymer. The research was conducted using single-crystal X-ray diffraction analysis and disclosed a complex architecture with a network of interatomic interactions (contribution 5).

Nascimento et al., described an interesting conversion of lupulone [9] into an annulated pyrazole through a hetero-cyclization reaction performed with phenylhydrazine. The structure of the obtained polycyclic heterocycle was ascertained through NMR spectroscopy (contribution 6).

Marzano et al., presented the structural analysis of a side product recovered during the attempts to alkylate the inosine N1 position regioselectively [10]. The N1-alkylated inosines were revealed to be fundamental building blocks for the preparation of cyclic inosine diphosphate ribose (cIDPR) analogs [11–13] to be exploited as potential intracellular Ca^{2+} ions mobilizers [14,15]. The side product was identified as an O6-alkylated inosine regioisomer through NMR analysis (contribution 7).

Amrane et al., treated 1-(4-chlorophenoxy)-4-methylphthalazine with the $PCl_5/POCl_3$ system to perform the $CH_3 \rightarrow CCl_3$ conversion. Unfortunately, a side dichloro methylphosphonic dichloride derivative was obtained as a single product (contribution 8).

A two-step conversion of natural betulin [16,17] to 19β,28-epoxy-18α-olean-3β-ol-2-furoate was realized by Lugemwa through a rearrangement in the E-ring followed by esterification on the A-ring of the obtained allobetulin (contribution 9).

Straniero et al. contributed to the Special Issue with three papers. In the first paper, the authors unexpectedly isolated (3-methylene-2,3-dihydronaphtho[2,3-*b*][1,4]dioxin-2-yl)methanol instead of the corresponding epoxide upon the exposition of 2,3-dihydronaphtho [1,4]dioxine-2-carbaldehyde to the Johnson–Corey–Chaykovsky reaction conditions [18] (contribution 10).

In the search for novel antimicrobial agents acting through the inhibition of the protein FtsZ [19], Straniero et al. also reported the synthesis and characterization of *threo* and *erythro* isomers of 6-fluoro-3-(2,3,6,7,8,9-hexahydronaphtho[2,3-*b*][1,4]dioxin-2-yl)-2,3-dihydrobenzo[*b*][1,4]dioxine-5-carboxamide, obtained as side products when the two isomers of the 2-(oxiran-2-yl)-2,3,6,7,8,9-hexahydronaphtho[2,3-*b*][1,4]dioxines were reacted with 2,6-difluorophenate (contribution 11).

Straniero et al., also found an unexpected conversion at room temperature of a pyridine derivative into the corresponding N-benzylated pyridinium salt and attributed the transformation to the presence of the unreacted benzyl bromide in the crude mixture (contribution 12).

The reaction of 3-methyl-2-thioxoimidazolidin-4-one with 1,3-dehydroadamantane afforded an unexpected side product, namely (*Z*)-2′-((adamantan-1-yl)thio)-1,1′-dimethyl-2′,3′-dihydro-[2,4′-biimidazolylidene]-4,5,5′(1*H*,1′*H*,3*H*)-trione, which was characterized by Burmistrov et al. via single-crystal X-ray diffraction analysis (contribution 13).

While searching for applications in small molecule activation reactions, a new binuclear manganese complex with two different N,O-ligands was synthesized and characterized by single-crystal X-ray diffraction analysis by Khrizanforova et al., (contribution 14). The authors found an interesting ligand environment in the crystal structure in the proximity of the two manganese centers.

Cely-Veloza et al. reported on a successful good-yielding microwave synthesis of a small series of diethyl 2-((arylamino)methylene)malonates, which were originally produced as side products of a three-component reaction (contribution 15). Interestingly, two compounds showed better IC_{50} than the positive control against the phytopathogens belonging to the family of *Fusarium oxysporum*.

In the paper published by Burcă et al., the authors explored the reactivity of triazoles, which are a class of five-membered heterocycles with remarkable biological properties [20]. In detail, they found that a new triazol-3-one unexpectedly formed following the reduction reaction of a heterocyclic thioketone with sodium borohydride in the presence of small amounts of water (contribution 16).

Aitken et al. characterized for the first time, through NMR and single-crystal X-ray diffraction experiments, a new dibromodisalicylaldehyde obtained as a side-product when studying the Baeyer–Villiger oxidation [21,22] of 5-bromo-2-methoxymethoxybenzaldehyde with *m*-chloroperoxybenzoic acid (contribution 17).

All the papers submitted to this Special Issue have been rigorously pre-checked by Guest Editors (GEs) before being sent for peer-review. The GEs especially thank the reviewers for verifying the correctness of the proposed side structures through a careful analysis of the experimental data reported in the manuscripts. It is pleasing to see that the acceptance rate for "Molecules from Side Reactions II" was 94%, which highlights the very high quality of research submitted to this Special Issue. Lastly, the GEs also wish to thank the Editor in Chief for accepting the Special Issue proposal and the Editorial Office staff for providing all the necessary assistance to carry out this project.

List of Contributions

1. Politano, F.; Brydon, W.P.; Nandi, J.; Leadbeater, N.E. Unexpected Metal-Free Dehydrogenation of a β-Ketoester to a Phenol Using a Recyclable Oxoammonium Salt. *Molbank* **2021**, *2021*, M1180. https://doi.org/10.3390/M1180.
2. Sepsey Für, C.; Keglevich, G.; Bölcskei, H. Unexpected Formation of 4-aryl-1-(Propane-2-ylidenehydrazono)-2,3-diazaspiro[5.5]undec-3-ene by the Reaction of Pyridazinethiones Derivatives with Hydrazine. *Molbank* **2021**, *2021*, M1243. https://doi.org/10.3390/M1243.
3. Rodríguez, R.; León, O.; Quiroga, F.; Cifuentes, J. *N*-{2-[(3-Oxo-1,3-dihydro-2-benzofuran-1-yl)acetyl]phenyl}acetamide. *Molbank* **2021**, *2021*, M1244. https://doi.org/10.3390/M1244.
4. Miyagawa, A.; Ohno, S.; Yamamura, H. *N,N*-Bis(hexyl α-D-acetylmannosyl) Acrylamide. *Molbank* **2021**, *2021*, M1255. https://doi.org/10.3390/M1255.
5. Rachid, L.N.; Corfield, P.W.R. Poly[3-methyl-1,3-oxazolidin-2-iminium[μ_3-cyanido-tri-μ_2-cyanido-κ^9C:N-tricuprate(I)]]. *Molbank* **2021**, *2021*, M1259. https://doi.org/10.3390/M1259.
6. Nascimento, J.E.R.d.; Hartwig, D.; Jacob, R.G.; Silva, M.S. 3-Isobutyl-5,5,7-tris(3-methylbut-2-en-1-yl)-1-phenyl-1,7-dihydro-4*H*-indazole-4,6(5*H*)-dione. *Molbank* **2022**, *2022*, M1330. https://doi.org/10.3390/M1330.

7. Marzano, M.; Terracciano, M.; Piccialli, V.; Mahal, A.; Nilo, R.; D'Errico, S. O6-[(2″,3″-*O*-Isopropylidene-5″-*O*-^{t}butyldimethylsilyl)pentyl]-5′-O-^{t}butyldiphenylsilyl-2′,3′-*O*-isopropylideneinosine. *Molbank* **2022**, *2022*, M1345. https://doi.org/10.3390/M1345.
8. Amrane, D.; Khoumeri, O.; Vanelle, P.; Primas, N. Dichloro{4-(4-chlorophenoxy)phthalazin-1-yl} methylphosphonic dichloride. *Molbank* **2022**, *2022*, M1439. https://doi.org/10.3390/M1439.
9. Lugemwa, F.N. 19β,28-Epoxy-18α-olean-3β-ol-2-furoate from Allobetulin (19β,28-Epoxy-18α-olean-3β-ol). *Molbank* **2022**, *2022*, M1499. https://doi.org/10.3390/M1499.
10. Suigo, L.; Lodigiani, G.; Straniero, V.; Valoti, E. (3-Methylene-2,3-dihydronaphtho[2,3-*b*][1,4]dioxin-2-yl)methanol. *Molbank* **2022**, *2022*, M1521. https://doi.org/10.3390/M1521.
11. Straniero, V.; Suigo, L.; Lodigiani, G.; Valoti, E. Obtainment of Threo and Erythro Isomers of the 6-Fluoro-3-(2,3,6,7,8,9-hexahydronaphtho[2,3-*b*][1,4]dioxin-2-yl)-2,3-dihydrobenzo[*b*][1,4]dioxine-5-carboxamide. *Molbank* **2023**, *2023*, M1559. https://doi.org/10.3390/M1559.
12. Suigo, L.; Straniero, V.; Valoti, E. 2-(1-Methoxycarbonyl-2-phenyleth-1-yl)-1-benzylpyridin-1-ium Bromide. *Molbank* **2023**, *2023*, M1738. https://doi.org/10.3390/M1738.
13. Burmistrov, V.; Mokhov, V.; Fayzullin, R.R.; Butov, G.M. (*Z*)-2′-((Adamantan-1-yl)thio)-1,1′-dimethyl-2′,3′-dihydro-[2,4′-biimidazolylidene]-4,5,5′(1*H*,1′*H*,3*H*)-trione. *Molbank* **2023**, *2023*, M1585. https://doi.org/10.3390/M1585.
14. Khrizanforova, V.V.; Fayzullin, R.R.; Budnikova, Y.H. Manganese(II) Bromide Coordination toward the Target Product and By-Product of the Condensation Reaction between 2-Picolylamine and Acenaphthenequinone. *Molbank* **2023**, *2023*, M1606. https://doi.org/10.3390/M1606.
15. Cely-Veloza, W.-F.; Quiroga, D.; Coy-Barrera, E. Diethyl 2-((aryl(alkyl)amino)methylene)malonates: Unreported Mycelial Growth Inhibitors against Fusarium oxysporum. *Molbank* **2023**, *2023*, M1630. https://doi.org/10.3390/M1630.
16. Burcă, I.; Badea, V.; Deleanu, C.; Bercean, V.; Péter, F. 4-(4-Ethoxyphenyl)-5-(4-methoxyphenyl)-2,4-dihydro-3*H*-1,2,4-triazol-3-one. *Molbank* **2023**, *2023*, M1705. https://doi.org/10.3390/M1705.
17. Aitken, R.A.; Cordes, D.; Ler, A.J.; McKay, A.P. 2,8-Dibromo-6*H*,12*H*-6,12-epoxydibenzo[*b*,*f*][1,5]dioxocine. *Molbank* **2023**, *2023*, M1729. https://doi.org/10.3390/M1729.

Author Contributions: Writing—original draft preparation, S.D. and A.G.; writing—review and editing, S.D. All authors have read and agreed to the published version of the manuscript.

Funding: This research received no external funding.

Acknowledgments: The authors are grateful to Luisa Cuorvo for her technical assistance.

Conflicts of Interest: The authors declare no conflict of interest.

References

1. Chen, Y.; Yan, B.; Cheng, Y. State-of-the-Art Review of Oxidative Dehydrogenation of Ethane to Ethylene over MoVNbTeOx Catalysts. *Catalysts* **2023**, *13*, 204. [CrossRef]
2. Miller, S.A.; Bobbitt, J.M.; Leadbeater, N.E. Oxidation of terminal diols using an oxoammonium salt: A systematic study. *Org. Biomol. Chem.* **2017**, *15*, 2817–2822. [CrossRef]
3. Neochoritis, C.G.; Zhao, T.; Dömling, A. Tetrazoles via Multicomponent Reactions. *Chem. Rev.* **2019**, *119*, 1970–2042. [CrossRef] [PubMed]
4. Huang, Z.; Meng, Y.; Wu, Y.; Song, C.; Chang, J. Synthesis of isoindolo[1,2-a]isoquinoline and isoindolo[2,1-a]quinoline derivatives via trifluoroacetic acid-mediated cascade reactions. *Tetrahedron* **2021**, *93*, 132280. [CrossRef]
5. Yadav, G.D.; Wagh, D.P. Claisen-Schmidt Condensation using Green Catalytic Processes: A Critical Review. *ChemistrySelect* **2020**, *5*, 9059–9085. [CrossRef]
6. Quintana, J.I.; Atxabal, U.; Unione, L.; Ardá, A.; Jiménez-Barbero, J. Exploring multivalent carbohydrate–protein interactions by NMR. *Chem. Soc. Rev.* **2023**, *52*, 1591–1613. [CrossRef]
7. Laigre, E.; Goyard, D.; Tiertant, C.; Dejeu, J.; Renaudet, O. The study of multivalent carbohydrate–protein interactions by bio-layer interferometry. *Org. Biomol. Chem.* **2018**, *16*, 8899–8903. [CrossRef]

8. Thalji, M.R.; Ibrahim, A.A.; Chong, K.F.; Soldatov, A.V.; Ali, G.A.M. Glycopolymer-Based Materials: Synthesis, Properties, and Biosensing Applications. *Top. Curr. Chem.* **2022**, *380*, 45. [CrossRef]
9. Carbone, K.; Gervasi, F. An Updated Review of the Genus Humulus: A Valuable Source of Bioactive Compounds for Health and Disease Prevention. *Plants* **2022**, *11*, 3434. [CrossRef] [PubMed]
10. Hyde, R.M.; Broom, A.D.; Buckheit, R.W. Antiviral Amphipathic Oligo- and Polyribonucleotides: Analogue Development and Biological Studies. *J. Med. Chem.* **2003**, *46*, 1878–1885. [CrossRef] [PubMed]
11. D'Errico, S.; Oliviero, G.; Borbone, N.; Amato, J.; Piccialli, V.; Varra, M.; Mayol, L.; Piccialli, G. Solid-Phase Synthesis of a New Diphosphate 5-Aminoimidazole-4-carboxamide Riboside (AICAR) Derivative and Studies toward Cyclic AICAR Diphosphate Ribose. *Molecules* **2011**, *16*, 8110–8118. [CrossRef]
12. Mahal, A.; D'Errico, S.; Borbone, N.; Pinto, B.; Secondo, A.; Costantino, V.; Tedeschi, V.; Oliviero, G.; Piccialli, V.; Piccialli, G. Synthesis of cyclic N 1 -pentylinosine phosphate, a new structurally reduced cADPR analogue with calcium-mobilizing activity on PC12 cells. *Beilstein J. Org. Chem.* **2015**, *11*, 2689–2695. [CrossRef] [PubMed]
13. D'Errico, S.; Greco, F.; Patrizia Falanga, A.; Tedeschi, V.; Piccialli, I.; Marzano, M.; Terracciano, M.; Secondo, A.; Roviello, G.N.; Oliviero, G.; et al. Probing the Ca^{2+} mobilizing properties on primary cortical neurons of a new stable cADPR mimic. *Bioorg. Chem.* **2021**, *117*, 105401. [CrossRef] [PubMed]
14. Bootman, M.D.; Collins, T.J.; Peppiatt, C.M.; Prothero, L.S.; MacKenzie, L.; De Smet, P.; Travers, M.; Tovey, S.C.; Seo, J.T.; Berridge, M.J.; et al. Calcium signalling—An overview. *Semin. Cell Dev. Biol.* **2001**, *12*, 3–10. [CrossRef]
15. Matikainen, N.; Pekkarinen, T.; Ryhänen, E.M.; Schalin-Jäntti, C. Physiology of Calcium Homeostasis. *Endocrinol. Metab. Clin. North Am.* **2021**, *50*, 575–590. [CrossRef] [PubMed]
16. Król, S.K.; Kiełbus, M.; Rivero-Müller, A.; Stepulak, A. Comprehensive Review on Betulin as a Potent Anticancer Agent. *BioMed Res. Int.* **2015**, *2015*, 584189. [CrossRef]
17. Lou, H.; Li, H.; Zhang, S.; Lu, H.; Chen, Q. A Review on Preparation of Betulinic Acid and Its Biological Activities. *Molecules* **2021**, *26*, 5583. [CrossRef]
18. Mondal, M.; Connolly, S.; Chen, S.; Mitra, S.; Kerrigan, N.J. Recent Developments in Stereoselective Reactions of Sulfonium Ylides. *Organics* **2022**, *3*, 320–363. [CrossRef]
19. Han, H.; Wang, Z.; Li, T.; Teng, D.; Mao, R.; Hao, Y.; Yang, N.; Wang, X.; Wang, J. Recent progress of bacterial FtsZ inhibitors with a focus on peptides. *FEBS J.* **2021**, *288*, 1091–1106. [CrossRef]
20. Gupta, O.; Pradhan, T.; Chawla, G. An updated review on diverse range of biological activities of 1,2,4-triazole derivatives: Insight into structure activity relationship. *J. Mol. Struct.* **2023**, *1274*, 134487. [CrossRef]
21. Renz, M.; Meunier, B. 100 Years of Baeyer–Villiger Oxidations. *Eur. J. Org. Chem.* **1999**, *1999*, 737–750. [CrossRef]
22. Sun, Y.; Hu, Z.; Peng, J.; Qin, Q.; Jiao, N. Alternative method to Baeyer–Villiger oxidation of cyclobutenones using I 2/DMSO catalytic systems. *Green Chem.* **2023**, *25*, 7079–7083. [CrossRef]

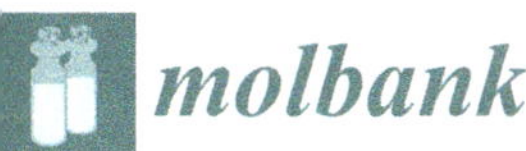

molbank

MDPI

Communication

Unexpected Metal-Free Dehydrogenation of a β-Ketoester to a Phenol Using a Recyclable Oxoammonium Salt

Fabrizio Politano, William P. Brydon, Jyoti Nandi and Nicholas E. Leadbeater *

Department of Chemistry, University of Connecticut, 55 North Eagleville Road, Storrs, CT 06269-3060, USA; fabrizio.politano@uconn.edu (F.P.); william.brydon@uconn.edu (W.P.B.); jyoti.nandi@uconn.edu (J.N.)

* Correspondence: nicholas.leadbeater@uconn.edu

Abstract: The conversion of ethyl 2-oxocyclohexanecarboxylate to ethyl salicylate using an oxoammonium salt is reported. The dehydrogenation reaction is operationally simple and compares favorably with previous literature examples for the same transformation and expands the scope of oxoammonium salts as reagents for oxidative functionalization processes.

Keywords: oxoammonium salt; dehydrogenation; phenol; recyclable; ketone

Citation: Politano, F.; Brydon, W.P.; Nandi, J.; Leadbeater, N.E. Unexpected Metal-Free Dehydrogenation of a β-Ketoester to a Phenol Using a Recyclable Oxoammonium Salt. *Molbank* **2021**, *2021*, M1180. https://doi.org/10.3390/M1180

Academic Editors: Stefano D'Errico and Annalisa Guaragna

Received: 23 December 2020
Accepted: 7 January 2021
Published: 13 January 2021

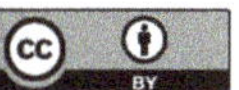

1. Introduction

Oxoammonium salts are stable, metal-free oxidants that are recyclable and can be used under mild conditions. They and their nitroxide analogs have been employed extensively for the oxidation of alcohols to aldehydes, ketones, and carboxylic acids [1–7]. The most widely used oxoammonium salt is 4-acetamido-2,2,6,6-tetramethylpiperidine-1-oxoammonium tetrafluoroborate, **1** (Figure 1) [7]. Moving beyond simple alcohol oxidation, **1** can also be used as a reagent for a range of oxidative functionalization reactions [8–11]. These include oxidative esterification [12], amidation [13], and the preparation of nitriles from aldehydes [14]. It is also possible to couple **1** with visible-light photocatalysis in a dual catalytic system [15–22]. When using **1** in a stoichiometric perspective, one transformation of particular interest is the dehydrogenation of ketones (Scheme 1) [23,24].

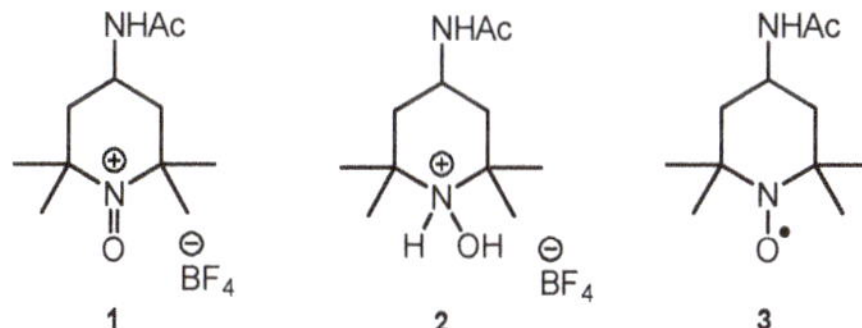

Figure 1. Oxoammonium salt **1** and its hydroxyammonium and nitroxide analogs **2**, and **3**.

3.8 eq. **1**
MeCN, 50 °C, 16 h
35-68%
R and R' = Me, allyl, propargyl, cyclohexenyl

2.4 eq. **1**
2.2 eq. 2,6-lutidine
CH_2Cl_2, Δ, 4-48 h
53-98%
R = aryl

Scheme 1. Dehydrogenation of ketones using oxoammonium salt **1**.

Ene-triketones have been prepared by oxidation of diketones [25], and perfluoroalkyl ketones can be converted to their α,β-unsaturated analogs [26]. Reactions are performed in the presence of a nitrogenous base such as pyridine or 2,6-dimethylpyridine (2,6-lutidine). A superstoichiometric quantity of the oxoammonium salt is required because, in the presence of a base, the hydroxyammonium byproduct, **2**, initially formed undergoes a comproportionation reaction with a further aliquot of **1** to generate two equivalents of nitroxide **3** [27,28]. Thus, a sacrificial equivalent of **1** is required in order to affect complete dehydrogenation of the substrate. The spent oxidant can be easily removed by filtration at the end of a reaction and converted back to **1** [29].

In an attempt to expand the scope of previous methodologies, we sought to use **1** for the dehydrogenation of a range of cyclohexanones. This transformation is traditionally performed using hypervalent iodine reagents [30] or by palladium catalysis [31]. We wanted to see if **1** could be used as an environmentally benign alternative. As a sharpening stone for probing this reaction, our attention focused on ethyl 2-oxocyclohexanecarboxylate, **4**, as a substrate. However, rather than obtaining ethyl 2-oxo-3-cyclohexene-1-carboxylate, **5**, as the product, we observed the formation of ethyl salicylate, **6**, a well-known phenolic compound (Scheme 2) [32–36]. We report this serendipitous discovery here.

1, 2,6-lutidine

MeCN, 50 °C, 96 h

4 — 5 EXPECTED — 6 OBSERVED

Scheme 2. Conversion of β-ketoester **4** to phenol **6** rather than α,β-unsaturated β-ketoester **5**.

2. Results and Discussion

Our discovery arose when we performed the reaction of **4** with 3.6 eq. of **1**, using 5 eq of 2,6-lutidine as a base. Heating an acetonitrile solution of the reagents at 50 °C for 96 h led to an almost equimolar ratio of phenol **6** and unreacted starting material **4** (Table 1, entry 1). Increasing the loading of **1** to 7.5 eq. and reducing the reaction time to 24 h, resulted in complete conversion to **6** (entry 2). Performing the reaction in absence of 2,6-lutidine was not successful, indicating the importance of the base (entry 3). Reducing the reaction temperature to 25 °C slowed the reaction considerably, it taking 72 h to reach completion (entries 4 and 5). Operating at 50 °C but reducing the oxoammonium salt loading to 5 eq required extending the reaction time to 72 h (entry 6). Attempts to perform the reaction catalytically in **1** using a number of secondary oxidants were not successful. In order to improve the efficacy of the stoichiometric protocol, we wanted to reduce the reaction time To achieve this, we turned to using microwave heating under sealed-vessel conditions as a tool. This way we were able to reach 100 °C simply and safely and could reduce the reaction time from 24 h to 30 min and obtain a near-quantitative conversion (entry 7). These became the optimal conditions for the protocol.

Our attention turned next to the isolation of the phenol from the product mixture With an organic base and byproducts from the oxoammonium salt in the mixture, isolation of **6** involved a series of extractions. The product mixture was first diluted with water and then dilute hydrochloric acid added. An extraction with petroleum ether removed non-acidic byproducts. The organic layer was then washed with dilute sodium hydroxide in order to extract the product as the phenoxide anion into the aqueous phase and leaving organic byproducts, spent oxidant, and any unreacted starting material in the organic phase. Acidification of the aqueous extract with dilute hydrochloric acid liberated the phenol which was then extracted using petroleum ether. Removal of the solvent gave **6** in 40% isolated yield.

Table 1. Optimization of reaction conditions for the conversion of β-ketoester **4** to phenol **6** [a].

Entry	1 (eq.)	2,6-Lutidine (eq.)	Temperature (°C)	Time (h)	Conversion to 6 (%) [b]
1	3.6	5	50	96	51
2	7.5	5	50	24	100
3	7.5	0	50	24	0
4	7.5	5	25	72	53
5	7.5	5	25	72	95
6	5.0	5	50	72	92
7 [c]	7.5	5	100	0.5	100

[a] Reagents and conditions: ethyl 2-oxocyclohexanecarboxylate (**4**, 0.5 mmol, 1 eq.), acetonitrile (2 mL, 0.25 M in **4**), requisite quantity of **1** and 2,6-lutidine, stirred at the desired temperature in an oil bath for the allotted time. [b] Determined using GCMS. [c] Performed using microwave heating.

The fact that phenol **6** is formed in the reaction of **4** with **1** is noteworthy in light of the two other literature reports of this transformation. One employs an *o*-iodoxybenzoic acid derivative bearing a trimethylammonium group [30]. A comparable yield of **6** is obtained in the oxidative dehydrogenation of **4**. The other approach involves the use of 10 mol% of palladium chloride in conjunction with 2 eq. of chloranil as a terminal oxidant [31]. The phenol product is obtained in 95% yield after 18 h. Compared to these reports, our methodology has the advantage that it is metal-free and that the oxidant is cheaper, easier to use, recyclable, and non-toxic.

3. Materials and Methods

3.1. General

All microwave-heating reactions were performed using a CEM Discover SP microwave unit (CEM Corporation, Matthews, NC, USA), in closed-vessel configuration. Temperature was measured by means of an IR temperature sensor located below the reaction vessel. NMR spectra (^{1}H, ^{13}C) were obtained in deuterated chloroform at 300 K using a Brüker DRX-400 400 MHz spectrometer (Brüker, Billerica, MA, USA). ^{1}H-NMR spectra were referenced to residual $CHCl_3$ (7.26 ppm) in $CDCl_3$. ^{13}C-NMR spectra were referenced to $CDCl_3$ (77.16 ppm). Reactions were monitored by an Agilent Technologies (Santa Clara, CA, USA) 7820A Gas Chromatograph attached to a 5975 Mass Spectrometer.

3.2. Chemicals

Ethyl 2-oxocyclohexanecarboxylate [CAS 1655-07-8] was purchased from Acros Organics (Geel, Belgium). 2,6-lutidine [CAS 108-48-5] was purchased from Oakwood Chemical (Estill, SC, USA). Acetonitrile [CAS 75-05-8] was obtained from Sigma-Aldrich (St. Louis, MO, USA). Petroleum ether [CAS 8032-32-4] was purchased from Fisher Scientific (Hampton, NH, USA). Deuterated chloroform ($CDCl_3$) [CAS 865-49-6] was purchased from Cambridge Isotope Laboratories (Tewksbury, MA, USA). Oxoammonium salt, **1**, [CAS 219543-09-6] was prepared using a literature procedure [29].

3.3. Synthesis of Ethyl Salicylate (**6**) *[CAS 118-61-6]*

Ethyl 2-oxocyclohexanecarboxylate [CAS 1655-07-8] (**4**, 1 mmol, 1 eq), 2,6-lutidine [CAS 108-48-5] (5 mmol, 5 eq), 4-acetylamino-2,2,6,6-tetramethylpiperidine-1-oxoammonium tetrafluoroborate (**1**, 7.5 mmol, 7.5 eq), acetonitrile (3 mL) and deionized water (1 mL) were added to a 40 mL-capacity glass tube equipped with a magnetic stir bar. The reaction mixture was sealed with a cap and placed into a CEM Discover SP microwave unit. The content of the vessel was heated to 100 °C and held at this temperature for 30 min, the microwave power automatically fluctuating to hold the reaction mixture at the desired temperature. The reaction mixture was stirred constantly. After the allotted time, the reaction mixture was allowed to cool to below 50 °C before taking the vessel out of the microwave unit. An intensely colored solution was obtained at this point. The product mixture was transferred from the glass tube to a separatory funnel whereupon water (2 mL) was added, followed by 1 M HCl (5 mL). An extraction with petroleum ether was performed (5 × 10 mL) in order to remove non-acidic byproducts. The organic layer was then washed with 0.5 M NaOH (2 × 25 mL) in order to extract the product in phenoxide anion form. At this point the color of the solution changed from yellow to green. The two basic aqueous fractions were collected and acidified with 2 M HCl until a pH of less than 3 was reached (~30 mL acid). At this point the solution turned a cloudy yellow color. This solution was extracted with petroleum ether (3 × 30 mL). The combined organic extracts were washed with brine (~30 mL) and dried over Na_2SO_4. The solvent was removed under reduced pressure by rotary evaporation affording pure phenol **6** as a yellow oil (66 mg, 40%). ^{1}H-NMR (400 MHz, $CDCl_3$): δ ppm 10.84 (s, 1H), 7.85 (dd, J = 8.0, 1.8 Hz, 1H), 7.45 (ddd, J = 8.8, 7.2, 1.8 Hz, 1H), 6.98 (dd, J = 8.4, 1.1 Hz, 1H), 6.88 (ddd, J = 8.2, 7.2, 1.1 Hz, 1H), 4.41 (q, J = 7.1 Hz, 2H), 1.42 (t, J = 7.1 Hz, 3H).^{13}C-NMR (101 MHz, $CDCl_3$): δ ppm 170.36, 161.83, 135.73, 130.05, 119.22, 117.70, 112.79, 77.48, 77.16, 76.84, 61.55, 14.33. GC-MS: (EI), m/z (relative intensity, %), 166 ($[M]^+$, 39), 121 (28), 120 (100), 92 (37), 65 (11). Spectral data for this compound are consistent with those previously reported [37,38] (Supplementary Materials).

4. Conclusions

In summary, we report the conversion of β-ketoester **4** to a phenol **6** using oxoammonium salt **1**. The reaction is operationally simple and compares favorably with previous literature examples for the same transformation. This serendipitous discovery opens the door to further exploration of the dehydrogenation of ketones to generate phenol products and work is currently underway in our laboratory to this end.

Supplementary Materials: The following are available online. ^{1}H- and ^{13}C-NMR, and GCMS spectra of product **6**.

Author Contributions: Conceptualization, N.E.L. and J.N.; methodology, W.P.B., J.N. and F.P.; data curation, W.P.B., J.N. and F.P.; writing—original draft preparation, N.E.L. and F.P.; writing—review and editing, W.P.B., N.E.L., J.N. and F.P.; supervision, N.E.L. and F.P.; project administration, N.E.L.; funding acquisition, N.E.L. All authors have read and agreed to the published version of the manuscript.

Funding: This research was funded by the University of Connecticut Research Enhancement Program and Office of Undergraduate Research.

Data Availability Statement: The data presented in this study are available in the article and Supplementary Material.

Acknowledgments: The University of Connecticut is thanked for financial support.

Conflicts of Interest: The authors declare no conflict of interest.

References

1. Shibuya, M. Nitroxyl Radical-Catalyzed Chemoselective Alcohol Oxidation for the Synthesis of Polyfunctional Molecules. *Tetrahedron Lett.* **2020**, *61*, 151515. [CrossRef]
2. Beejapur, H.A.; Zhang, Q.; Hu, K.; Zhu, L.; Wang, J.; Ye, Z. TEMPO in Chemical Transformations: From Homogeneous to Heterogeneous. *ACS Catal.* **2019**, *9*, 2777–2830. [CrossRef]
3. Tebben, L.; Studer, A. Nitroxides: Applications in synthesis and in polymer chemistry. *Angew. Chem. Int. Ed.* **2011**, *50*, 5034–5068. [CrossRef] [PubMed]
4. Ciriminna, R.; Pagliaro, M. Industrial oxidations with organocatalyst TEMPO and its derivatives. *Org. Proc. Res. Dev.* **2010**, *14*, 245–251. [CrossRef]
5. Bobbitt, J.M.; Brückner, C.; Merbouh, N. Oxoammonium-catalyzed oxidation. *Org. React.* **2009**, *74*, 103–206.
6. Vogler, T.; Studer, A. Applications of TEMPO in Synthesis. *Synthesis* **2008**, 1979–1993. [CrossRef]
7. Kelly, C.B. 2,2,6,6-Tetramethylpiperidine-Based Oxoammonium Salts. *Synlett* **2013**, *24*, 527–528. [CrossRef]
8. Leadbeater, N.E.; Bobbitt, J.M. TEMPO-Derived Oxoammonium Salts as Versatile Oxidizing Agents. *Aldrichimica Acta* **2014**, *47*, 65–74.
9. Gini, A.; Brandhofer, T.; Mancheño, O.G. Recent Progress in Mild Csp3-H Bond Dehydrogenative or (Mono-) Oxidative Functionalization. *Org. Biomol. Chem.* **2017**, *15*, 1294–1312. [CrossRef]

10. Garcia-Mancheño, O.; Stopka, T. TEMPO Derivatives as Alternative Mild Oxidants in Carbon–Carbon Coupling Reactions. *Synthesis* **2013**, *45*, 1602–1611. [CrossRef]
11. Rohlmann, R.; Garcia-Mancheño, O. Metal-Free Oxidative C(sp^3)-H Bond Couplings as Valuable Synthetic Tools for C–C Bond Formations. *Synlett* **2013**, *24*, 6–10. [CrossRef]
12. Kelly, C.B.; Mercadante, M.A.; Wiles, R.J.; Leadbeater, N.E. Oxidative Esterification of Aldehydes Using a Recyclable Oxoammonium Salt. *Org. Lett.* **2013**, *15*, 2222–2225. [CrossRef] [PubMed]
13. Ovian, J.M.; Kelly, C.B.; Pistritto, V.A.; Leadbeater, N.E. Accessing N-Acyl Azoles via Oxoammonium Salt-Mediated Oxidative Amidation. *Org. Lett.* **2017**, *19*, 1286–1289. [CrossRef] [PubMed]
14. Kelly, C.B.; Lambert, K.M.; Mercadante, M.A.; Ovian, J.M.; Bailey, W.F.; Leadbeater, N.E. Access to Nitriles from Aldehydes Mediated by an Oxoammonium Salt. *Angew. Chem. Int. Ed.* **2015**, *54*, 4241–4245. [CrossRef]
15. Twilton, J.; Le, C.; Zhang, P.; Shaw, M.H.; Evans, R.W.; MacMillan, D.W.C. The merger of transition metal and photocatalysis. *Nat. Rev. Chem.* **2017**, *1*, 52. [CrossRef]
16. Shaw, M.H.; Twilton, J.; Macmillan, D.W.C. Photoredox Catalysis in Organic Chemistry. *J. Org. Chem.* **2016**, *81*, 6898–6926. [CrossRef]
17. Romero, N.A.; Nicewicz, D.A. Organic Photoredox Catalysis. *Chem. Rev.* **2016**, *116*, 10075–10166. [CrossRef]
18. Prier, C.K.; Rankic, D.A.; Macmillan, D.W.C. Visible Light Photoredox Catalysis with Transition Metal Complexes: Applications in Organic Synthesis. *Chem. Rev.* **2013**, *113*, 5322–5363. [CrossRef]
19. Nandi, J.; Vaughan, M.Z.; Sandoval, A.L.; Paolillo, J.M.; Leadbeater, N.E. Oxidative Amidation of Amines in Tandem with Transamidation: A Route to Amides Using Visible-Light Energy. *J. Org. Chem.* **2020**, *85*, 9219–9229. [CrossRef]
20. Nandi, J.; Leadbeater, N.E. Visible-light-driven catalytic oxidation of aldehydes and alcohols to nitriles by 4-acetamido-tempo using ammonium carbamate as a nitrogen source. *Org. Biomol. Chem.* **2019**, *17*, 9182–9186. [CrossRef]
21. Nandi, J.; Witko, M.L.; Leadbeater, N.E. Combining Oxoammonium Cation Mediated Oxidation and Photoredox Catalysis for the Conversion of Aldehydes into Nitriles. *Synlett* **2018**, *29*, 2185–2190.
22. Pistritto, V.A.; Paolillo, J.M.; Bisset, K.A.; Leadbeater, N.E. Oxidation of α-trifluoromethyl and non-fluorinated alcohols via the merger of oxoammonium cations and photoredox catalysis. *Org. Biomol. Chem.* **2018**, *16*, 4715–4719. [CrossRef] [PubMed]
23. Bosque, I.; Chinchilla, R.; Gonzalez-Gomez, J.C.; Guijarro, D.; Alonso, F. Cross-Dehydrogenative Coupling Involving Benzylic and Allylic C-H Bonds. *Org. Chem. Front.* **2020**, *7*, 1717–1742. [CrossRef]
24. Bao, X.; Jiang, W.; Liang, J.; Huo, C. One-Electron Oxidative Dehydrogenative Annulation and Cyclization Reactions. *Org. Chem. Front.* **2020**, *7*, 2107–2144. [CrossRef]
25. Eddy, N.A.; Kelly, C.B.; Mercadante, M.A.; Leadbeater, N.E.; Fenteany, G. Access to dienophilic ene-triketone synthons by oxidation of diketones with an oxoammonium salt. *Org. Lett.* **2012**, *14*, 498–501. [CrossRef]
26. Hamlin, T.A.; Kelly, C.B.; Leadbeater, N.E. Dehydrogenation of Perfluoroalkyl Ketones Using a Recyclable Oxoammonium Salt. *Eur. J. Org. Chem.* **2013**, 3658–3661. [CrossRef]
27. Hamlin, T.A.; Kelly, C.B.; Ovian, J.M.; Wiles, R.J.; Tilley, L.J.; Leadbeater, N.E. Toward a Unified Mechanism for Oxoammonium Salt-Mediated Oxidation Reactions: A Theoretical and Experimental Study Using a Hydride Transfer Model. *J. Org. Chem.* **2015**, *80*, 8150–8167. [CrossRef]
28. Bobbitt, J.M.; Bartelson, A.L.; Bailey, W.F.; Hamlin, T.A.; Kelly, C.B. Oxoammonium Salt Oxidations of Alcohols in the Presence of Pyridine Bases. *J. Org. Chem.* **2014**, *79*, 1055–1067. [CrossRef]
29. Mercadante, M.; Kelly, C.B.; Bobbitt, J.M.; Tilley, L.J.; Leadbeater, N.E. Synthesis of 4-acetamido-2,2,6,6-tetramethylpiperidine-1-oxoammonium tetrafluoroborate and 4-acetamido-(2,2,6,6-tetramethyl-piperidin-1-yl)oxyl and their use in oxidative reactions. *Nat. Protoc.* **2013**, *8*, 666–676. [CrossRef]
30. Cui, L.Q.; Dong, Z.L.; Liu, K.; Zhang, C. Design, Synthesis, Structure, and Dehydrogenation Reactivity of a Water Soluble o-Iodoxybenzoic Acid Derivative Bearing a Trimethylammonium Group. *Org. Lett.* **2011**, *13*, 6488–6491. [CrossRef]
31. Samadi, S.; Orellana, A. A New Route to Phenols: Palladium-Catalyzed Cyclization and Oxidation of γ,δ-Unsaturated Ketones. *ChemCatChem* **2016**, *8*, 2472–2475. [CrossRef]
32. Zhao, L.; Huang, G.; Guo, B.; Xu, L.; Chen, J.; Cao, W.; Zhao, G.; Wu, X. Diastereo- and Enantioselective Propargylation of Benzofuranones Catalyzed by Pybox-Copper Complex. *Org. Lett.* **2014**, *16*, 5584–5587. [CrossRef] [PubMed]
33. Shome, S.; Singh, S.P. Design and synthesis of ruthenium bipyridine catalyst: An approach towards low-cost hydroxylation of arenes and heteroarenes. *Tetrahedron Lett.* **2017**, *58*, 3743–3746. [CrossRef]
34. Bayguzina, A.R.; Tarisova, L.I.; Khusnutdinov, R.I. Synthesis of Hydroxybenzoic Acids and Their Esters by Reaction of Phenols with Carbon Tetrachloride and Alcohols in the Presence of Iron Catalysts. *Russ. J. Gen. Chem.* **2018**, *88*, 208–215. [CrossRef]
35. Gopinath, R.; Barkakaty, B.; Talukdar, B.; Patel, B.K. Peroxovanadium-Catalyzed Oxidative Esterification of Aldehydes. *J. Org. Chem.* **2003**, *68*, 2944–2947. [CrossRef]
36. Brenner, J.E. The Synthesis of 2-Carboethoxy-Δ^2-cyclohexenone. *J. Org. Chem.* **1961**, *26*, 22–27. [CrossRef]
37. Magano, J.; Chen, M.H.; Clark, J.D.; Nussbaumer, T. 2-(Diethylamino)ethanethiol, a New Reagent for the Odorless Deprotection of Aromatic Methyl Ethers. *J. Org. Chem.* **2006**, *71*, 7103–7105. [CrossRef]
38. Parkins, M.V.; Kitching, W.; Drew, R.A.I.; Moore, C.J.; König, W.A. Chemistry of fruit flies: Composition of the male rectal gland secretions of some species of South-East Asian Dacinae. Re-examination of *Dacus cucurbitae* (melon fly). *J. Chem. Soc. Perkin Trans.* **1990**, *1*, 1111–1117.

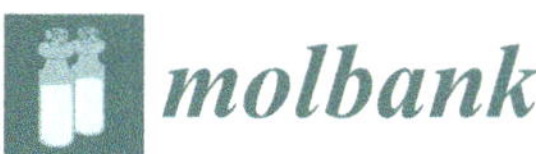
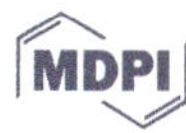

Communication

Unexpected Formation of 4-aryl-1-(Propane-2-ylidenehydrazono)-2,3-diazaspiro[5.5]undec-3-ene by the Reaction of Pyridazinethiones Derivatives with Hydrazine

Csilla Sepsey Für, György Keglevich and Hedvig Bölcskei *

Department of Organic Chemistry and Technology, Budapest University of Technology and Economics, 1111 Budapest, Hungary; sepsey.fur.csilla@vbk.bme.hu (C.S.F.); keglevich.gyorgy@vbk.bme.hu (G.K.)
* Correspondence: bolcskei.hedvig@vbk.bme.hu; Tel.: +36-1-463-2208

Abstract: After making a new series of spiro[cycloalkane]pyridazinones with high Fsp^3 character available, the new target was to synthesize derivatives comprising nitrogen-containing heterocycles, such as triazolo or tetrazolo rings. The corresponding thioxo derivatives (**1a**,**b**) seemed to be good starting materials for the synthesis of tetrazolo derivatives. The reaction of the pyridazinethiones (**1a**,**b**) with hydrazine surprisingly resulted in Schiff bases (**3a**,**b**) deriving from the reaction of hydrazones (**2a**,**b**) with acetone.

Keywords: pyridazinethione; spiro[cycloalkane]pyridazine; hydrazine; acetone; Schiff base

Citation: Sepsey Für, C.; Keglevich, G.; Bölcskei, H. Unexpected Formation of 4-aryl-1-(Propane-2-ylidenehydrazono)-2,3-diazaspiro[5.5]undec-3-ene by the Reaction of Pyridazinethiones Derivatives with Hydrazine. *Molbank* **2021**, *2021*, M1243. https://doi.org/10.3390/M1243

Academic Editors: Stefano D'Errico and Annalisa Guaragna

Received: 26 May 2021
Accepted: 15 June 2021
Published: 2 July 2021

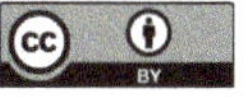

1. Introduction

The molecule bank of a company might play an important role in the early phase of preclinical drug discovery. To find a hit, a high-throughput screening (HTS) campaign may be a useful tool [1]. In the design of new compounds for a molecule bank, the application of some widely used rules (Lipinski rule of five, Veber's rule) [2–4] and other concepts of medicinal chemistry, such as the role of aromatic rings or bioisosteric nitrogen-containing heterocycles, are of key importance [5–8]. Lovering introduced the Fsp^3 character, which usually shows a good correlation with logP and other physicochemical parameters [9,10]. With the consideration of the above aspects, a series of spiro[cycloalkane]pyridazinones with high Fsp^3 character and advantageous physicochemical parameters was synthetized [11–13]. Starting from 2-oxaspiro[4.4]nonane-1,3-dione and 2-oxaspiro[4.5]-1,3-dione, the ketocarboxylic acids were obtained by Friedel-Crafts or Grignard reaction. The ring closure took place with hydrazine or its derivatives: methylhydrazine and phenylhydrazine. A few of the obtained dihydropyridazine derivatives were alkylated. The corresponding pyridazinonethiones (**1**) were prepared by the reaction of pyridazinones with phosphorus pentasulfide [14] (Scheme 1).

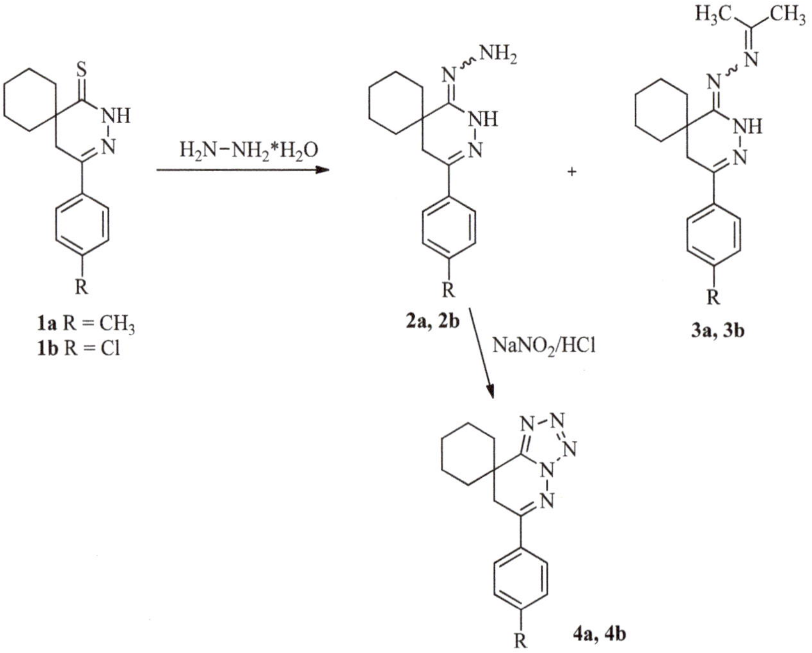

Scheme 1. Synthesis of hydrazone and tetrazolo derivatives starting from spiro[cycloalkane]pyridazinethiones.

2. Results and Discussion

We wanted to extend this compound family with further examples, combining the spiro[cycloalkane]pyridazines with nitrogen-containing heterocycles, such as triazole or tetrazole. The hydrazone derivatives of **1a,b** may be important intermediates for the synthesis of tetrazoles. To obtain these compounds, the reaction of pyridazinethiones (**1a** and **1b**) with hydrazine in tetrahydrofuran was studied [14]. In the case of the chloro and methyl derivatives, the *E* and *Z* stereoisomers of the desired hydrazones (**2a** (R = CH_3, yield: 59%) and **2b** (R = Cl, yield:61%)) were obtained surprisingly with a small amount of a side product (**3a** and **3b**), which is the Schiff base of the expected hydrazones with acetone (**3a,b**). The structures of the isolated by-products were established by detailed ^{1}H and ^{13}C NMR and HRMS studies. The hydrazones (**2a** R = CH_3 and **2b** R = Cl) might have been the intermediates, which reacted with the trace amount of acetone present in the glassware. Reacting the hydrazones (**2a** R = CH_3 and **2b** R = Cl) with sodium nitrite, the corresponding tetrazole derivatives (**4a** R = CH_3 and **4b** R = Cl) were obtained smoothly [14]. According to the database SciFinder, the compounds **3a** and **3b** (R = CH_3, Cl) are new compounds, which may be valuable members of a molecule bank. Table 1 summarizes the most important physicochemical parameters of **3a,b**. Interestingly the Fsp^3 character of compounds **3a,b** is high, but the logP and clogP values (4.6–5.2) are not advantageous enough.

Table 1. The physicochemical parameters of the hydrazone derivatives.

Starting Material	R^1	Product	Fsp^3	LogP	ClogP	TPSA
1a	CH_3	**3a**	0.53	4.59	5.03	49.11
1b	Cl	**3b**	0.50	4.66	5.24	49.11

3. Materials and Methods

3.1. General Information, TLC, Preparative TLC

Hydrazine hydrate [10217-52-4], tetrahydrofuran [109-99-9], dichloromethane [75-09-2], heptane [142-82-5], methanol [67-56-1] were purchased from SigmaAldrich. TLC was carried out using Kieselgel 60 F_{254} (Merck 1.05554.0001). The analytical samples for NMR and HRMS studies were purified by preparative TLC using Kieselgel 60 F_{254} (Merck 1.07748.1000) coated glass plates.

3.2. NMR Spectroscopy

NMR measurements were performed on a Varian VNMRS 400 MHz NMR spectrometer equipped with a ^{15}N-^{31}P{^{1}H-^{19}F} 5 mm OneNMR room temperature probe, a Varian VNMRS 500 MHz NMR spectrometer equipped with a ^{1}H {^{13}C/^{15}N} 5 mm PFG Triple Resonance ^{13}C Enhanced Cold Probe, a Varian VNMRS 800 MHz NMR spectrometer equipped with a ^{1}H{^{13}C/^{15}N} TripleResonance^{13}C Enhanced Salt Tolerant Cold Probe (Varian, Inc., Palo Alto, CA, USA), a Bruker Avance III HDX 500 MHz NMR spectrometer equipped with a ^{1}H {^{13}C/^{15}N} 5 mm TCI CryoProbe, and a Bruker Avance III HDX 500 MHz NMR spectrometer equipped with a ^{1}H-^{19}F{^{13}C/^{15}N} 5 mm TCI CryoProbe (Bruker Corporation, Billerica, MA, USA). ^{1}H and ^{13}C chemical shifts are given on the delta scale as parts per million (ppm) with tetramethylsilane (TMS) (^{1}H, ^{13}C) or dimethylsulfoxide-d_6(^{13}C) as the internal standard (0.00 ppm and 39.4 ppm, respectively). ^{1}H-^{1}H, direct ^{1}H-^{13}C, and long-range ^{1}H-^{13}C scalar spin–spin connectivity were established from 2D COSY, TOCSY, HSQC, and HMBC experiments. ^{1}H-^{1}H spatial proximities were determined using two-dimensional NOESY or ROESY experiments. ^{15}N Chemical shifts are referenced to nitromethane (0.0 ppm) and are obtained from ^{1}H-^{15}N HMBC measurements. All pulse sequences were applied by using the standard spectrometer software package. All experiments were performed at 298 K. NMR spectra were processed using VnmrJ 2.2 Revision C (Varian, Inc. Palo Alto, CA, USA), Bruker TopSpin 3.5 pl 6 (Bruker Corporation, Billerica, MA, USA), and ACD/Spectrus Processor version 2017.1.3 (Advanced Chemistry Development, Inc., Toronto, ON, Canada).

3.3. Mass Spectrometry

HRMS and MS-MS analyses were performed on a ThermoVelos Pro Orbitrap Elite (Thermo Fisher Scientific) system. The ionization method was ESI operated in positive ion mode. The protonated molecular ion peaks were fragmented by CID at a normalized collision energy of 35%. For the CID experiment, helium was used as the collision gas. The samples were dissolved in methanol. Data acquisition and analysis were accomplished with Xcalibur software version 2.0 (Thermo Fisher Scientific, Waltham, MA, USA).

3.4. General Procedure for the Preparation of 1-(Propane-2-ylidenehydrazono)-4-(p-substituted phenyl)-2,3-diazaspiro[5.5]undec-3-ene (3a,3b)

The hydrazine monohydrate (0.10 mL, 1.2 mmol) was dissolved in THF (5 mL), and then the corresponding pyridazinethione derivatives (**1a,b**) (0.40 mmol) were also dissolved in THF (15 mL) and added dropwise to the hydrazine solution. The reaction mixture was stirred at reflux for 12 h, and then the solvent was evaporated. The residue was dissolved in dichloromethane (20 mL) and washed with distilled water (2 × 10 mL). The organic layer was dried over $MgSO_4$, filtered and evaporated. The crude productwas purified by preparative thin-layer chromatography (eluent: heptane:dichloromethane:methanol/5:5:1) to give by-products and hydrazone derivatives.

1-(Propan-2-ylidenehydrazono)-4-(p-tolyl)-2,3-diazaspiro[5.5]undec-3-ene (**3a**) Yield: 14%;Rf(heptane:dichloromethane:methanol/5:5:1) = 0.48,^{1}H NMR (499.9 MHz; DMSO-d_6) δ = 1.31–1.71 (m, 10H, cyclohexyl); 1.94 (s, 3H, H-3′); 1.97 (s, 3H, H-1′); 2.37 (s, 3H, C(4″)-CH_3); 2.72 (s, 2H, H-5); 7.22 (m, 2H, H-3″, H-5″); 7.67 (m, 2H, H-2″, H-6″); 9.75 (br s, 1H, NH-2) ppm; ^{13}C NMR (125.7 MHz; DMSO-d_6) δ = 17.52 (C-3′); 20.72 (C-4″-CH3); 20.97 (C-8, C-10); 25.51 (C-9); 27.77 (C-1′); 30.75 (C-5); 32.75 (C-7, C-11); 33.31 (C-6); 124.88

(C-2″, C-6″); 128.98 (C-3″, C-5″); 134.32 (C-1″); 134.32 (C-4″); 145.67 (C-4); 153.55 (C-1), 160.79 (C-2′) ppm; ^{15}N NMR (40.5 MHz; DMSO-d_6) δ = −333.48 (N-2′); −306.25 (N-3), −145.69 (N-2); (N-1) ppm; HRMS: M + H = 311.22313 (delta = 0.3 ppm; $C_{19}H_{27}N_4$). MS-MS (CID = 35%; rel. int. %): 282(100); 267(31); 255(13); 239(24); 227(8); 212(39); 199(10); 186(3), 138(2).

4-(4-Chlorophenyl)-1-(propan-2-ylidenehydrazono)-2,3-diazaspiro[5.5]undec-3-ene (**3b**) Yield: 7%; ^{1}H NMR (499.9 MHz; DMSO-d_6) δ = 1.31–1.71 (m, 10H, cyclohexyl); 1.94 (s, 3H, H-3′); 1.97 (s, 3H, H-1′); 2.74 (s, 2H, H-5); 7.46 (m, 2H, H-3″, H-5″); 7.80 (m, 2H, H-2″, H-6″); 9.90 (s, 1H, NH-2) ppm; ^{13}C NMR (125.7 MHz; DMSO-d_6) δ = 17.55 (C-3′); 20.93 (C-8, C-10); 24.77 (C-1′); 25.50 (C-9); 30.68 (C-5); 32.78 (C-7, C-11); 33.20 (C-6); 126.65 (C-2″, C-6″); 128.40 (C-3″, C-5″); 133.00 (C-4″); 135.93 (C-1″); 144.31 (C-4); 153.10 (C-1), 161.10 (C-2′) ppm; ^{15}N NMR (40.5 MHz; DMSO-d_6) δ = −333.80 (N-2′); −309.88 (N-3); −267.65 (N-1′); −147.14 (N-2) ppm; HRMS: M + H = 331.16715 (delta = −3.8 ppm; $C_{18}H_{24}N_4Cl$) HR-ESI-MS-MS (CID = 45%; rel. int. %): 302(100); 301(17); 287(30); 275(10); 261(12); 259(17), 247(10); 232(33).

4. Conclusions

Reacting spiro[cycloalkane]pyridazinethiones with hydrazine in tetrahydrofuran, the desired hydrazones and, surprisingly, their Schiff bases with acetone were obtained. The hydrazones might have reacted with the acetone present in the glassware. The structures of the isolated *p*-substituted 4-aryl-1-(propane-2-ylidenehydrazono)-2,3- diazaspiro[5.5]undec-3-enes (**3a**,**3b**) have been fully characterized by ^{1}H, ^{13}C, ^{15}N NMR and HRMS.

Supplementary Materials: The following are available online: HRMS, ^{1}H, and ^{13}C NMR spectra of **3a**,**b**

Author Contributions: C.S.F. and H.B. planned the experiments. C.S.F. carried out the experimental work. H.B. managed the project and wrote the paper. G.K. was the consultant. All authors have read and agreed to the published version of the manuscript.

Funding: C.S.F. is grateful for the support of the Gedeon Richter's Centenárium Foundation.

Institutional Review Board Statement: Not applicable.

Informed Consent Statement: Not applicable.

Data Availability Statement: The data presented in this study are available within the article or supplementary material.

Acknowledgments: The authors are grateful to Áron Szigetvári for the NMR and Miklós Dékány for the HRMS studies.

Conflicts of Interest: The authors declare no conflict of interest.

References

1. Inglese, J.; Auld, D.S. Application of High Throughput Screening (HTS) Techniques: Overview of Applications in Chemical Biology. *Wiley Encycl. Chem. Biol.* **2009**, *2*, 260–274. [CrossRef]
2. Lipinski, C.A.; Lombardo, F.; Dominy, B.W.; Feeney, P.J. Experimental and computational approaches to estimate solubility and permeability in drug discovery and development settings. *Adv. Drug Deliv. Rev.* **1997**, *23*, 3–25. [CrossRef]
3. Lipinski, C.A. Lead- and drug-like compounds: The rule-of-five revolution. *Drug Discov. Today Technol.* **2004**, *1*, 337–341 [CrossRef] [PubMed]
4. Veber, D.F.; Johnson, S.R.; Cheng, H.-Y.; Smith, B.R.; Ward, K.W.; Kopple, K.D. Molecular Properties That Influence the Oral Bioavailability of Drug Candidates. *J. Med. Chem.* **2002**, *45*, 2615–2623. [CrossRef] [PubMed]
5. Ritchie, T.; Macdonald, S.J. The impact of aromatic ring count on compound developability—are too many aromatic rings a liability in drug design? *Drug Discov. Today* **2009**, *14*, 1011–1020. [CrossRef] [PubMed]
6. Ritchie, T.J.; Macdonald, S.J.; Young, R.J.; Pickett, S.D. The impact of aromatic ring count on compound developability: Further insights by examining carbo- and hetero-aromatic and -aliphatic ring types. *Drug Discov. Today* **2011**, *16*, 164–171. [CrossRef] [PubMed]
7. Ritchie, T.J.; Macdonald, S.J.F. Physicochemical Descriptors of Aromatic Character and Their Use in Drug Discovery. *J. Med. Chem* **2014**, *57*, 7206–7215. [CrossRef] [PubMed]
8. Wermuth, C.G. Are pyridazines privileged structures? *Med. Chem. Comm.* **2011**, *2*, 935–941. [CrossRef]

9. Lovering, F.; Bikker, J.; Humblet, C. Escape from Flatland: Increasing Saturation as an Approach to Improving Clinical Success. *J. Med. Chem.* **2009**, *52*, 6752–6756. [CrossRef] [PubMed]
10. Lovering, F. Escape from Flatland 2: Complexity and promiscuity. *Med. Chem. Comm.* **2013**, *4*, 515–519. [CrossRef]
11. Für, C.S.; Riszter, G.; Gerencsér, J.; Szigetvári, Á.; Dékány, M.; Hazai, L.; Keglevich, G.; Bölcskei, H. Synthesis of Spiro[cycloalkane-pyridazinones] with High Fsp3 Character. *Lett. Drug Des. Discov.* **2020**, *17*, 731–744. [CrossRef]
12. Für, C.S.; Horváth, E.J.; Szigetvári, Á.; Dékány, M.; Hazai, L.; Keglevich, G.; Bölcskei, H. Synthesis of Spiro[cycloalkane-pyridazinones] with High Fsp3 Character Part 2*. *Lett. Org. Chem.* **2021**, *18*, 373–381. [CrossRef]
13. Für, C.S.; Bölcskei, H. New Spiro[cycloalkane-pyridazinone] Derivatives with Favorable Fsp^3 Character. *Chemistry* **2020**, *2*, 837–848. [CrossRef]
14. Für, C.S.; Riszter, G.; Szigetvári, Á.; Dékány, M.; Keglevich, G.; HazaI, L.; Bölcskei, H. Novel Ring Systems: Spiro[Cycloalkane] Derivatives of Triazolo- and Tetrazolo-Pyridazines. *Molecules* **2021**, *26*, 2140. [CrossRef]

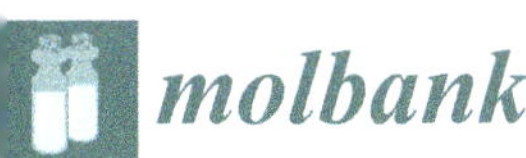

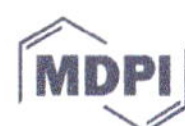

Short Note

N-{2-[(3-Oxo-1,3-dihydro-2-benzofuran-1-yl)acetyl]phenyl}acetamide

Ricaurte Rodríguez *, Omar León, Felipe Quiroga and Jonnathan Cifuentes

Investigation Group in Heterocyclic Chemistry, Chemistry Department, Universidad Nacional de Colombia-Sede Bogotá, Carrera 30, Calle 45-03, Bogotá 111321, Colombia; omleonr@unal.edu.co (O.L.); juquirogas@unal.edu.co (F.Q.); jcifuentesh@unal.edu.co (J.C.)

* Correspondence: rrodrigueza@unal.edu.co; Tel.: +57-1-316-5000 (ext. 14458)

Abstract: With the aim of obtaining different derivatives belonging to the isoindolo[2,1-*a*]quinoline family, we have synthesized a novel *N*-{2-[(3-oxo-1,3-dihydro-2-benzofuran-1-yl)acetyl]phenyl}acetamide derivative by a Claisen–Smichdt-type condensation reaction in 75% yield.

Keywords: phthalides; isobenzofuranones; Fischer indole synthesis; Claisen–Schmidt reaction; Witkop reaction

Citation: Rodríguez, R.; León, O.; Quiroga, F.; Cifuentes, J. N-{2-[(3-Oxo-1,3-dihydro-2-benzofuran-1-yl)acetyl]phenyl}acetamide. *Molbank* **2021**, *2021*, M1244. https://doi.org/10.3390/M1244

Academic Editors: Stefano D'Errico and Annalisa Guaragna

Received: 5 June 2021
Accepted: 22 June 2021
Published: 2 July 2021

Publisher's Note: MDPI stays neutral with regard to jurisdictional claims in published maps and institutional affiliations.

1. Introduction

2-Benzofuran-1(3*H*)-ones or isobenzofuranones (also known as phthalides) are considered privileged scaffolds, owing to their wide range of biological properties. More precisely, some phthalide derivatives have been evaluated as antioxidant **1** [1], anti-HIV-1 **2** [2], antileishmanial **3** [3] and antifungal **4** [4] while other phthalides are known for their herbicidal properties **5** [5] (Figure 1).

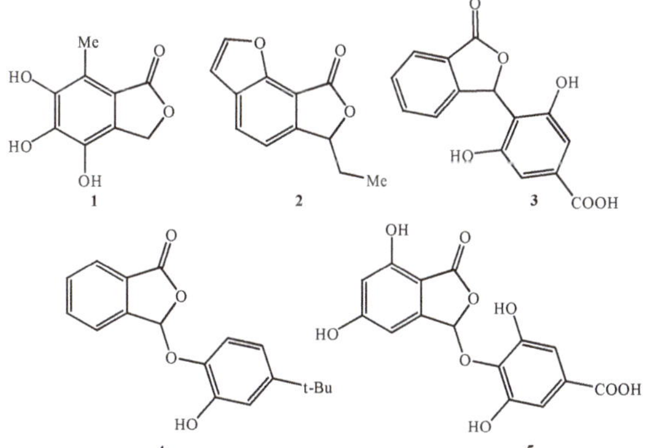

Figure 1. Some examples of phthalide derivatives with outstanding biological activities.

Additionally, phthalide derivatives are important intermediates in the synthesis of other relevant heterocyclic systems, as is the case for 2,3-dihydro-1*H*-isoindol-1-one derivatives, which are another type of unique molecules [6–9] (Scheme 1).

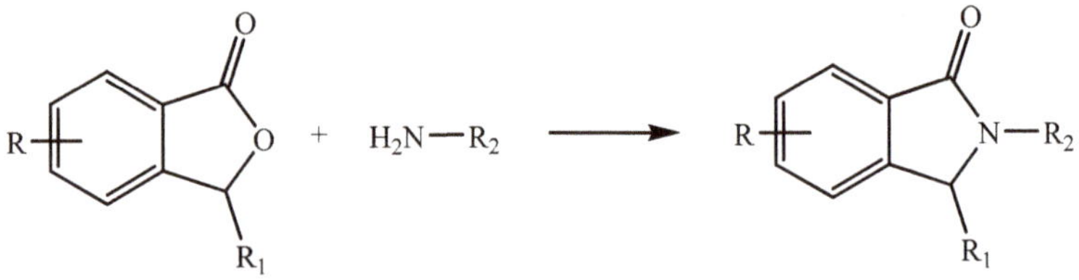

R= H, Br, Cl, OMe; R_1= Ph, indol-3-yl; R_2= Ph, 4-$MeOC_6H_4$, pyridin-2-yl

6 7 8

Scheme 1. Synthesis of 2,3-dihydro-1*H*-isoindol-1-one derivatives **8** from pthalides **6**.

Herein, we carried out the synthesis of a phtalide derivatives based on a Claisen-Smichdt reaction. We surmise that the novel synthetic route proposed could be exploited for the generation of new compounds that belong to the isoindolo[2,1-*a*]quinoline scaffold **9** (Figure 2).

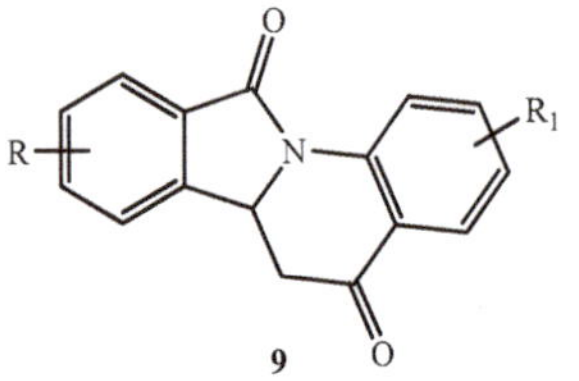

Figure 2. General structure of the target isoindolo[2,1-*a*]quinoline derivatives.

2. Results and Discussion

The synthesis of isoindolo[2,1-*a*]quinoline derivatives **9** (Figure 2) was based on a first condensation step to obtain product **12** as the key intermediate, mediated by the Claisen–Schmidt reaction as depicted in Scheme 2.

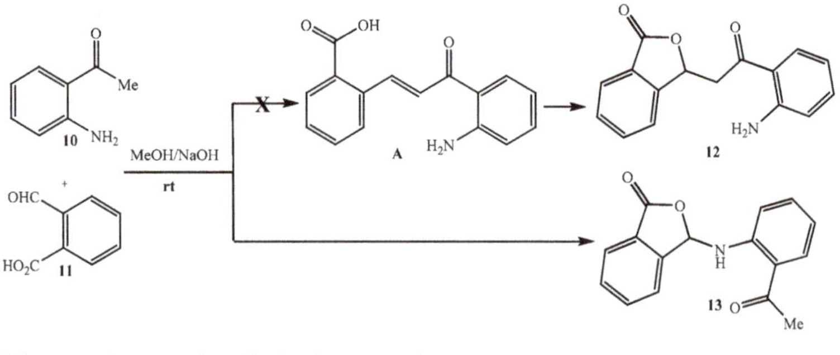

Scheme 2. Attempt of synthesis of compound **12**.

However, we were not able to isolate intermediate 12. Instead, we obtained byproduct **13**. Normally, compounds such as **12** are obtained in basic or neutral conditions, in a good yield [10–14]. Therefore, chalcone **A** should be presumably an intermediate in the synthesis of compound **12**.

In order to overcome the aforementioned drawback, we proposed a new synthetic route which began with the preparation of 2,3-dimethylindole (**14**) using a Fischer indole methodology. Then, the indole **14** was oxidized with a Witkop oxidation reaction to yield 2-(*N*-acetyl)acetophenone derivative **15** in an 80% yield. Finally, the Claisen–Schmidt type reaction between **15** and aldehyde **11** (Scheme 3) generated compound **16** (*N*-acetyl derivative of intermediate **12**) in a remarkable 75% yield.

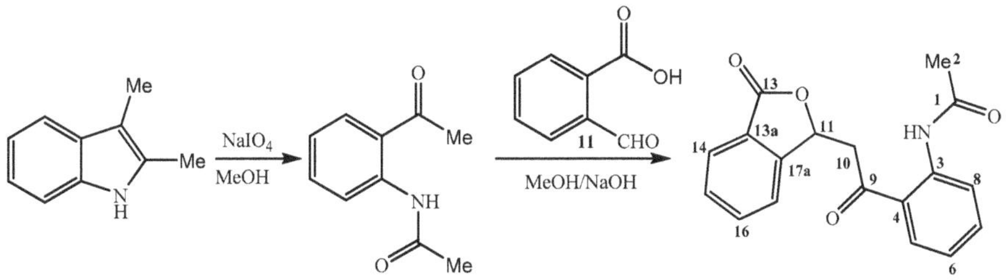

Scheme 3. Synthetic sequence for the target N-acetyl derivative **16**.

Compound **16** was characterized by a set of high resolution analytical techniques (IR, NMR, MS) and by its melting point. In the IR spectrum, at 3313 cm^{-1} an absorption band corresponding to N-H of the N-acetylated group was observed. At 1764 cm^{-1} a strong absorption band was assigned to the lactone carbonyl group. Another characteristic signal found at 1692 cm^{-1} was assigned to the ketone carbonyl group. Finally, the absorption bands attributed to the C-O and C-N bonds appeared around 1018 cm^{-1} and 1232 cm^{-1}. The high-resolution mass spectrum of compound **16** featured an ion peak at m/z = 332.08905 that is in accordance with the $[M + Na]^+$ molecular ion. The spectrum also revealed the presence of two peaks at m/z = 310.10700 and 348.06267, attributed to ions $[M + H]^+$ and $[M + K]^+$, respectively.

The ^1H NMR spectrum (Supplementary Materials) of the pure compound showed a set of signals that was in accordance with the proposed structure. Thus, the firs signal encountered at 11.07 ppm was attributed to NH proton. In the low-field region, we detected three doublets resonating at 8.22, 7.96 and 7.86 ppm that were assigned to protons H-14, H-5 and H-17, respectively. Two broad signals centered at 7.78 and 7.61 ppm were attributed to protons H-7, H-8, H-15 and H-16, respectively. The more shielded aromatic proton H-6 resonates as a triplet centered at 7.19 ppm. Three sets of signals, which are related to an ABX system, appear centered at 6.10, 3.85 and 3.70 ppm, respectively. These signals were assigned to H-11 (H_X) and H-10 (H_A and H_B). Finally, in the high-field region of the spectrum, we observed only the presence of a singlet, centered at 2.14 ppm, that corresponded to the methyl group of the N-acetyl portion (H-2).

Additionally, in the ^{13}C NMR spectrum, we observed a total of 18 signals. These findings are further supported by the APT experiment, in which seven signals for quaternary carbons were observed (in agreement with the proposed structure): three belonging to the carbonyl groups at 200.4 (C-9), 169.9 (C-13) and 169.0 (C-1) ppm, while the others corresponded to aromatic carbons. In addition, in the high-field region we observed the presence of a signal resonating at 44.4 ppm that was primarily attributed to the CH_2 (C-10) carbon (methylene and quaternary carbons appear in negative phase in the APT spectrum). All these findings are in agreement with the proposed structure for compound **16**.

In conclusion, we developed a three-step synthetic strategy which comprises a Fischer indole synthesis, a Witkop indole oxidation and a Claisen–Schmidt condensation reaction to obtain phthalide **16**. We envisage that this synthetic route can prove useful for the preparation of isoindolo[2,1-*a*]quinoline **9** derivatives.

3. Materials and Methods

3.1. General Information

Reagents and solvents used were obtained from commercial sources and were used without previous purification. The reaction progress was monitored by TLC with 0.2 mm precoated plates of silica gel 60 F254 (Merck). The melting point was measured using a Stuart SMP3 melting point apparatus (Cole-Parmer, Staffordshire, UK) and is uncorrected. The IR spectrum was recorded on a Shimadzu IR Affinity (Shimadzu, Kyoto, Japan) with ATR probe. The ^1H and ^{13}C-NMR spectra were recorded in a BRUKER DPX 400 spectrophotometer (Bruker, Bruker BioSpin GmbH, Rheinstetten, Germany) operating at 400 and 100 MHz, respectively, using DMSO-d_6 as the solvent. Chemical shifts (δ) are given in ppm and coupling constants (J) are given in *Hz*. The following abbreviations are used for multiplicities: s = singlet, d = doublet, t = triplet, dd = doublet of doublets, and m = multiplet. The mass spectrum was acquired on a SHIMADZU Quadrupole Time-of-Flight Liquid Chromatograph Mass Spectrometer (Q-TOF LCMS-9030 using the Nexera Mikros).

3.2. *Synthesis of N-{2-[(3-Oxo-1,3-dihydro-2-benzofuran-1-yl)acetyl]phenyl}acetamide* **16**

A mixture of 2-formylbenzoic acid (2 mmol) and NaOH (4 mmol) was dissolved in 10 mL of MeOH. The mixture was stirred for 5 min at room temperature, then compound **15** (2 mmol) was added. The reaction was stirred at 20 °C for 12 h (TLC control). At the end, the reaction mixture was neutralized with AcOH and poured into 40 mL of water. The obtained solid was collected and washed with cold acetone yielding compound **16** as a beige solid.

Yield: 464 mg, 75%. R_f = 0.28 (Hexane:Ethyl acetate (6:4)). M.p. 171–173 °C. FT-IR (KBr disk) (cm^{-1}): 3313 (NH), 2921 (aliphatic CH), 1764, 1692, 1648 (C=O). ^{1}H NMR (400 MHz, DMSO-d_6) δ (ppm) 2.14 (s, 3H, CH_3), 3.70 (dd, J = 7.7 Hz, 1H), 3.85 (dd, J = 6.7 Hz, 1H), 6.10 (dd, 1H), 7.19 (t, J = 7.6 Hz, 1H), 7.58–7.64 (m, J = 7.3 Hz, 1H, H-4), 7.74–7.82 (m, J = 7.3 Hz, 1H), 7.86 (d, J = 7.9 Hz, 2H), 7.96 (d, J = 7.7 Hz, 2H), 8.22 (d, J = 8.0 Hz, 1H), 11.07 (s, 1H, NH). ^{13}C NMR (100 MHz, DMSO-d_6) δ (ppm) 24.7 (C-2), 44.4 (C-10), 77.2 (C-11), 121.2 (CH), 123.0 (CH), 123.2 (CH), 124.8 (C-17a), 125.0 (C-5), 125.5 (C-3), 129.4 (CH), 130.8 (CH), 134.3 (CH), 134.4 (CH), 138.8 (C-13a), 149.8 (C-4), 169.0 (C-1), 169.9 (C-13), 200.4 (C-9). HR-MS (ESI^+): m/z calculated for $[M + H]^+$: 310.10738, found: 310.10700; calculated for $[M + Na]^+$: 332.08988, found: 332.08905 and calculated for: $[M + K]^+$: 348.06382, found: m/z: 348.06267.

Supplementary Materials: The following materials: Figure S1. ^{1}H-NMR spectrum for compound **16**, Figure S2. ^{13}C-NMR spectrum for compound **16**, Figure S3. APT spectrum for compound **16**, Figure S4. High Resolution Mass Spectrum for compound **16** and Figure S5. FT-IR spectrum for compound **16**.

Author Contributions: The authors R.R., O.L., F.Q. and J.C. designed and accomplished the research. They also analyzed the data and wrote the paper together. Finally, all authors have read and agreed to the published version of the manuscript.

Funding: This research received no external funding.

Institutional Review Board Statement: Not applicable.

Informed Consent Statement: Not applicable.

Data Availability Statement: The data presented in this study are available in this article.

Acknowledgments: The authors wish to thank the Universidad Nacional de Colombia-Sede Bogotá and Dirección de Investigación y Extensión, Sede Bogotá for financial support. Authors thank Rodrigo Abonia, Paula J. Celis-Salazar and Andres Felipe Sierra for reviewing the present manuscript.

Conflicts of Interest: The authors declare no conflict of interest.

References

1. Zou, S.; Wang, Z.; Wang, J.; Wei, G.; Wang, W.; Zang, Y.; Zeng, F.; Chen, K.; Liu, J.; Wang, J.; et al. Five new aza-epicoccone derivatives from Aspergillus flavipes. *Fitoterapia* **2018**, *124*, 127–131. [CrossRef] [PubMed]
2. Qin, X.-D.; Dong, Z.-J.; Liu, J.-K.; Yang, L.-M.; Wang, R.-R.; Zheng, Y.-T.; Lu, Y.; Wu, Y.-S.; Zheng, Q.-T. Concentricolide, an anti-HIV agent from the ascomycete Daldinia concentrica. *Helv. Chim. Acta* **2006**, *89*, 127–133. [CrossRef]
3. Rodrigues, M.P.; Tomaz, D.C.; de Souza, L.Â.; Onofre, T.S.; de Menezes, W.A.; Almeida, J.; Suarez, A.M.; de Almeida, M.R.; da Silva, A.M.; Costa, G.; et al. Synthesis of cinnamic acid derivatives and leishmanicidal activity against Leishmania braziliensis. *Eur. J. Med. Chem.* **2019**, *183*, 111688. [CrossRef] [PubMed]
4. Fan, L.; Luo, B.; Luo, Z.; Zhang, L.; Fan, J.W.; Tang, L.; Li, Y. Synthesis and antifungal activities of 3-substituted phthalide derivatives. *Z. Naturforsch. B* **2019**, *74*, 811–818. [CrossRef]
5. Teixeira, R.R.; Pereira, W.L.; Tomaz, D.C.; de Oliveira, F.M.; Giberti, S.; Forlani, G. Synthetic analogues of the natural com-pound cryphonectric acid interfere with photosynthetic machinery through two different mechanisms. *J. Agric. Food Chem.* **2013**, *61*, 5540–5549. [CrossRef] [PubMed]

6. Zhang, S.; Shi, X.; Li, J.; Hou, Z.; Song, Z.; Su, X.; Peng, D.; Wang, F.; Yu, Y.; Zhao, G. Nickel-catalized amidoalkylation reaction of γ-hidroxy lactams: An access to 3-substituted isoindolinones. *ACS Omega* **2019**, *4*, 19420–19436. [CrossRef] [PubMed]
7. Sashidhara, K.V.; Singh, L.R.; Palnati, G.R.; Avula, S.R.; Kant, R. A catalyst-free one pot protocol for the construction of sub-stituted isoindolinones under sustainable conditions. *Synlett* **2016**, *27*, 2384–2390. [CrossRef]
8. Lübbers, T.; Angehrn, P.; Gmünder, H.; Herzig, S. Design, synthesis, and structure-activity relationship studies of new phenolic DNA gyrase inhibitors. *Bioorg. Med. Chem. Lett.* **2007**, *17*, 4708–4714. [CrossRef] [PubMed]
9. Bassin, J.P.; Anagani, B.; Benham, C.; Goyal, M.; Hashemian, M.; Gerhard, U. Synthesis and spectral characterization of ben-zo-[6,7][1,5]diazocino[2,1-a]isoindol-12-(14H)-one derivatives. *Molecules* **2016**, *21*, 967. [CrossRef] [PubMed]
10. Abonia, R.; Cuervo, P.; Insuasty, B.; Quiroga, J.; Nogueras, M.; Cobo, J.; Meier, H.; Lotero, E. An Amberlyst-15®Mediated Synthesis of New Functionalized Dioxoloquinolinone Derivatives. *TOOCJ* **2008**, *2*, 26–34. [CrossRef]
11. Lee, J.; Jung, H. An Efficient Synthesis of 2,3-Dihydro-2-phenyl-4-quinolones from 2′-Aminoacetophenones. *J. Korean Chem. Soc.* **2007**, *51*, 106–110. [CrossRef]
12. Yaeghoobi, M.; Frimayanti, N.; Chee, C.F.; Ikram, K.K.; Najjar, B.O.; Zain, S.M.; Abdullah, Z.; Wahab, H.; Rahman, N.A. QSAR, in silico docking and in vitro evaluation of chalcone derivatives as potential inhibitors for H1N1 virus neuraminidase. *Med. Chem. Res.* **2016**, *25*, 2133–2142. [CrossRef]
13. Pan, G.F.; Su, L.; Zhang, Y.L.; Guo, S.H.; Wang, Y.Q. Organocatalytic one-pot asymmetric synthesis of 2-aryl-2,3-dihydro-4-quinolones. *RSC Adv.* **2016**, *6*, 25375–25378. [CrossRef]
14. Ullah, A.; Ansari, F.L.; ul-Haq, I.; Nazir, S.; Mirza, B. Combinatorial synthesis, lead identification, and antitumor study of a chalcone-based positional-scanning library. *Chem. Biodivers.* **2007**, *4*, 203–214. [CrossRef]

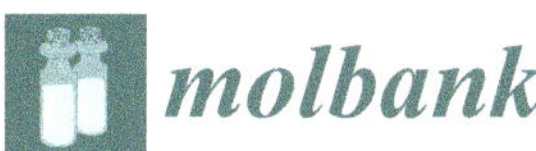 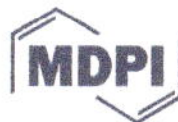

Short Note

N,*N*-Bis(hexyl α-D-acetylmannosyl) Acrylamide

Atsushi Miyagawa *, Shinya Ohno and Hatsuo Yamamura

Department of Materials Science and Engineering, Nagoya Institute of Technology, Gokiso, Showa-ku, Nagoya 466-8555, Japan; s.ohno.145@nitech.ac.jp (S.O.); yamamura.hatsuo@nitech.ac.jp (H.Y.)
* Correspondence: miyagawa.atsushi@nitech.ac.jp; Tel.: +81-52-735-5239

Abstract: Glycosyl monomers for the assembly of multivalent ligands are typically synthesized using carbohydrates with biological functions and polymerizable functional groups such as acrylamide or styrene introduced into the carbohydrate aglycon, and monomers polymerized using a radical initiator. Herein, we report the acryloylation of 6-aminohexyl α-D-mannoside and its conversion into the glycosyl monomer bearing an acrylamide group. The general acryloylation procedure afforded the desired *N*-hexyl α-D-acetylmannosyl acrylamide monomer as well as an unexpected compound with a close R_f value. The compounds were separated and analyzed by nuclear magnetic resonance spectroscopy and mass spectrometry, which revealed the unknown compound to be the bivalent *N*,*N*-bis(hexyl α-D-acetylmannosyl) acrylamide monomer, which contains two hexyl mannose units and one acrylamide group. To the best of our knowledge, this side reaction has not previously been disclosed, and may be useful for the construction of multivalent sugar ligands.

Keywords: glycosyl monomer; acryloylation; acrylamide; glycopolymer; bivalent ligand

Citation: Miyagawa, A.; Ohno, S.; Yamamura, H. *N*,*N*-Bis(hexyl α-D-acetylmannosyl) Acrylamide. *Molbank* **2021**, *2021*, M1255. https://doi.org/10.3390/M1255

Academic Editors: Stefano D'Errico and Annalisa Guaragna

Received: 7 June 2021
Accepted: 20 July 2021
Published: 22 July 2021

1. Introduction

Many biological events in organisms are associated with carbohydrates on cell surfaces [1–4]. Carbohydrates assemble into clusters in raft domains and on polysaccharides and proteins to acquire high affinities for carbohydrate-binding proteins (CBMs). The clusters, as multivalent ligands, interact with CBMs to induce biological events [5–7]. Multivalency, which is important for carbohydrate–protein interactions, has also been imitated by synthetic polymers that contain carbohydrates; this affinity-enhancing effect of a multivalent ligand is known as the "cluster effect". The polymer generally contains carbohydrates with pendants on the polymer back bones, which are generally chosen to be acrylamide [8,9], styrene [10,11], or norbornene [12,13]. A polymerizable carbohydrate monomer consists of a carbohydrate, a linker, and a polymerizable functional group. Carbohydrates include monosaccharides as well as oligosaccharides as ligands. The linker controls the flexibility and the binding space in the carbohydrate—protein interaction, while polymerizable functional groups modulate solubility and polymer structure, and these units are chosen to suit the research purpose. Studies into the preparation of glycomonomers and glycopolymers has continued to date with the aim of clarifying the biological mechanism and applying them to devices and biomaterials [14–17].

In this study, a mannosyl monomer was prepared using a general method in which 6-aminohexyl α-D-acetylmannoside was acryloylated to afford *N*-hexyl α-D-acetylmannosyl acrylamide. Surprisingly, a previously undocumented side-reaction was observed during acryloylation, the product of which was separated by silica-gel column chromatography and identified by nuclear magnetic resonance (NMR) spectroscopy and mass spectrometry (MS) to be *N*,*N*-bis(hexyl α-D-acetylmannosyl) acrylamide, which is a bivalent monomer containing two mannose residues. The discovery of this unusual bivalent monomer is described herein.

2. Results and Discussion

6-Aminohexyl α-D-mannoside (**1**) was prepared from D-mannose in five steps, which included acetylation, 1-deactylation, introduction of the trichloroacetimidate, glycosylation with 6-aminohexan-1-ol, and deacetylation. Mannoside (**1**) was converted into a mannosyl monomer bearing an acrylamide group by treatment with acryloyl chloride and sodium carbonate in methanol at 0 °C for 13 h, followed by acetylation (Scheme 1). The reaction mixture was evaporated and separated by silica-gel chromatography to provide two compounds that were subjected to NMR spectroscopy (Figures S1 and S2) and matrix assisted laser desorption ionization-time of flight (MALDI-TOF) MS (Figure S3). Their ^{1}H NMR spectra showed similar peaks; however, integration of the sugar and alkyl peaks of the compound of higher R_f revealed the presence of two 6-aminohexyl α-D-mannoside units per acryloyl group. Furthermore, the amide peak was absent in the NMR spectrum of this compound (Figure 1). In the IR spectrum, the N–H stretching vibration was also not observed (Figure S4). The mass spectrum of this unknown compound is displayed in Figure 2.

1. Acryloyl chloride, Na_2CO_3 MeOH, 0 °C, 13 h
2. Ac_2O, Pyridine, r.t., 20 h

1 → **2** (35 %) + **3** (26 %)

Scheme 1. Acryloylation of 6-aminohexyl α-D-mannside (**1**).

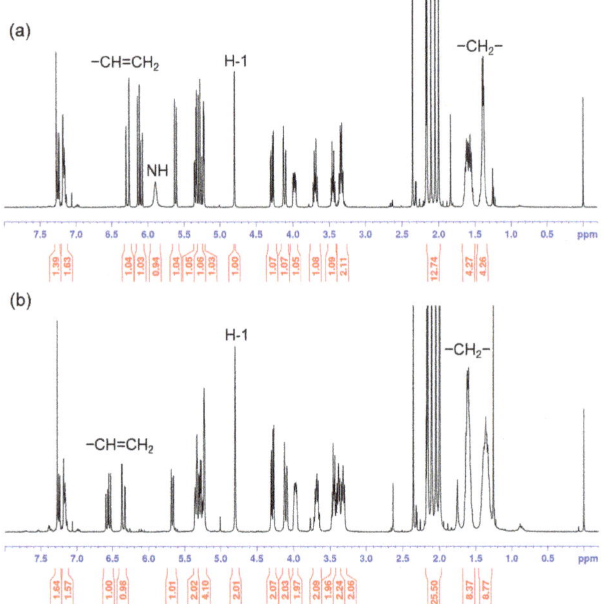

Figure 1. ^{1}H NMR spectra of (**a**) *N*-hexyl α-D-acetylmannosyl acrylamide (**2**) and (**b**) *N*,*N*-bis(hexyl α-D-acetylmannosyl) acrylamide (**3**).

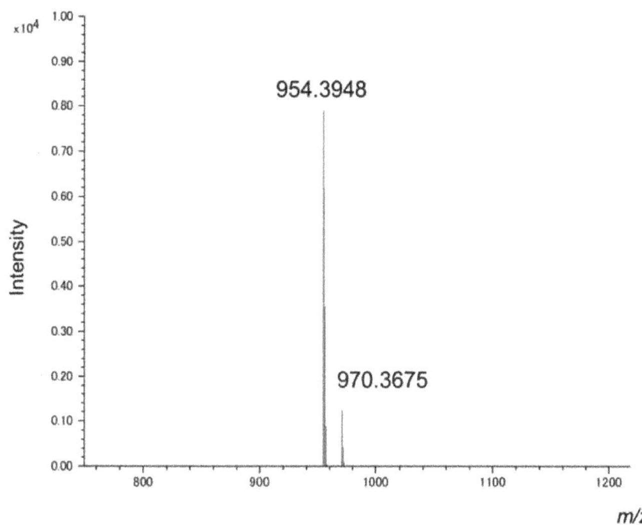

Figure 2. MALDI-TOF mass spectrum of *N,N*-bis(hexyl α-D-acetylmannosyl) acrylamide (**3**).

The above-mentioned results suggest that the unexpected compound contains two hexyl mannose units and one acryloyl group, from which we concluded that the acryloylation of **1** gave *N*-hexyl α-D-acetylmannosyl acrylamide (**2**) and *N,N*-bis(hexyl α-D-acetylmannosyl) acrylamide (**3**), which were isolated as pure syrups in yields of 35% and 26%, respectively, along with a considerable amount of a mixture of the two. It is interesting to note that the analogous side reaction that forms the bisamide was not observed in the case of 2-aminoethyl α-D-mannoside and the acryloylation for *N*-hexyl α-D-acetylmannosyl acrylamide (**2**). Therefore, *N,N*-bis(hexyl α-D-acetylmannosyl) acrylamide (**3**) was given only in the acryloylation for 6-aminohexyl α-D-mannoside (**1**). To the best of our knowledge, this is the first report of such a side reaction using the general acryloylation procedure. While the reaction mechanism is not clear, the bivalent monomer bearing the two sugar units may be useful for the preparation of multivalent glycopolymers.

3. Materials and Methods

3.1. General

All reagents were purchased from FUJIFILM Wako Pure Chemical Corporation (Osaka, Japan). Methanol was prepared by storage over molecular sieves (3Å) that were activated under vacuum at 200 °C. Analytical thin-layer chromatography (TLC) was performed using Merck silica gel 60 F_{254} plates (layer thickness: 0.25 mm, Darmstadt, Germany). TLC plates were dipped in 85:10:5 (*v*/*v*/*v*) methanol/resorcinol/concentrated sulfuric acid and/or 0.7% ninhydrin/ethanol, followed by heating for a few minutes for visualization purposes. Column chromatography was performed using silica gel (Silica gel 60 N, spherical neutral, particle size 63–210 µm, Kanto Chemical, Tokyo, Japan). ^{1}H and ^{13}C NMR spectra were acquired on an AVANCE 400 Plus spectrometer (Bruker, Rheinstetten, Germany) in chloroform-*d* and reported in δ relative to tetramethylsilane (0.00 ppm for ^{1}H and 77.0 ppm for ^{13}C). MALDI-TOF mass spectra were recorded on a Jeol JMS-S3000 spectrometer (Tokyo, Japan) using 2,5-dihydroxybenzoic acid as the matrix. The Fourier transform infrared (FTIR) spectra were measured on a Jasco FT-IR 4100 spectrometer (Tokyo, Japan) and reported as wavenumber (cm^{-1}). Pellet samples for FTIR were fabricated using KBr.

3.2. Acryloylation of 6-Aminohexyl α-D-Mannside (1)

6-Aminohexyl α-D-mannside **1** (976 mg, 3.13 mmol) was dissolved in methanol (21.0 mL). Sodium carbonate was added to the solution and the mixture was stirred at 0 °C, after which acryloyl chloride (380 μL, 4.70 mmol) was slowly added dropwise over 10 min and then stirred at 0 °C for 13 h. The mixture was evaporated and acetic anhydride (11.0 mL, 117 mmol) and pyridine (11.0 mL, 136 mmol) were added at room temperature, stirred for 20 h, and then evaporated. The residue was extracted with chloroform and washed successively with aqueous 1 M hydrochloric acid, aqueous sodium hydrogen carbonate, and brine, dried over anhydrous sodium sulfate, filtered, and then evaporated. The residue was purified by silica gel chromatography three times using 5:1 (*v*/*v*) toluene/acetone as the eluent to give **2** (553 mg, 35%), **3** (391 mg, 26%), and a mixture of **2** and **3** (231 mg; **2**:**3** = 2.7:1).

Analytical data for **2**. R_f 0.54 (toluene/acetone, 1:1); ^{1}H NMR (400 MHz, $CDCl_3$) δ 6.28 (dd, $J_{\text{-CH=,Htrans}}$ = 16.4 Hz, $J_{\text{Htrans,Hcis}}$ = 1.6 Hz, 1 H, =CH_{trans}H), 6.11 (dd, $J_{\text{-CH=,Hcis}}$ = 10.4 Hz, 1 H, =C*H*−), 5.90 (s, 1 H, N*H*), 5.62 (dd, 1 H, =CHH_{cis}), 5.34 (dd, $J_{2,3}$ = 3.6 Hz, $J_{3,4}$ = 10.0 Hz, 1 H, H-3), 5.28 (dd, $J_{4,5}$ = 19.8 Hz, 1 H, H-4), 5.22 (dt, $J_{1,2}$ = 1.6 Hz, 1 H, H-2), 4.80 (d, 1 H, H-1), 4.28 (dd, $J_{5,6a}$ = 5.6 Hz, $J_{6a,6b}$ = 12.2 Hz, 1 H, H-6a), 4.11 (dd, $J_{5,6b}$ = 2.4 Hz, 1 H, H-6b), 3.98 (dt, 1 H, H-5), 3.69 (dt, $J_{\text{OCHa, 2CH2}}$ = 9.6 Hz, $J_{\text{OCHa, OCHb}}$ = 6.4 Hz, 1 H, −OCH_aH$_b$−), 3.45 (dt, $J_{\text{OCHa, 2CH2}}$ = 6.4 Hz, 1 H, −OCH$_a$$H_b$−), 3.33 (dq, $J_{\text{CHaNH, CHbNH}}$ = 3.2 Hz, $J_{\text{CH2NH, 5CH2}}$ = 7.2 Hz, 2 H, −CH_2NH−), 2.16 (s, 3 H, COCH_3), 2.11 (s, 3 H, COCH_3), 2.05 (s, 3 H, COCH_3), 2.00 (s, 3 H, COCH_3), 1.65–1.53 (m, 4 H, ^{2}CH_2, ^{5}CH_2), 1.43–1.38 (m, 4 H, ^{3}CH_2, ^{4}CH_2); ^{13}C NMR (101 MHz, $CDCl_3$) δ 170.6, 170.1, 170.0, 169.7, 165.5, 130.9, 129.0 (toluene), 128.2 (toluene), 125.2 (toluene), 126.0, 97.5, 69.6, 69.1, 68.4, 66.2, 62.5, 39.4, 30.9 (toluene), 29.4, 29.0, 26.6, 25.9, 20.8, 20.7, 20.7.

Analytical data for **3**. R_f 0.64 (toluene/acetone, 1:1); ^{1}H NMR (400 MHz, $CDCl_3$) δ 6.55 (dd, $J_{\text{-CH=,Htrans}}$ = 16.8 Hz, $J_{\text{Htrans,Hcis}}$ = 2.4 Hz, 1 H, =CH_{trans}H), 6.35 (dd, $J_{\text{-CH=,Hcis}}$ = 10.4 Hz, 1 H, =C*H*−), 5.68 (dd, 1 H, =CHH_{cis}), 5.36–5.22 (m, 6 H, H-2, H-3, H-4), 4.80 (s, 2 H, H-1), 4.30 (dd, $J_{5,6a}$ = 5.2 Hz, $J_{6a,6b}$ = 12.0 Hz, 2 H, H-6a), 4.11 (d, 2 H, H-6b), 3.97 (dt, 2 H, H-5), 3.68 (dt, $J_{\text{OCHa, 2CH2}}$ = 9.6 Hz, $J_{\text{OCHa, OCHb}}$ = 6.8 Hz, 2 H, −OCH_aH$_b$−), 3.48–3.30 (m, 6 H, −OCH$_a$$H_b$−, −C$H_2$NH-), 2.16 (s, 6 H, COC$H_3$), 2.11 (s, 6 H, COC$H_3$), 2.05 (s, 6 H, COC$H_3$), 2.00 (s, 6 H, COC$H_3$), 1.63–1.60 (m, 8 H, ^{2}CH_2, ^{5}CH_2), 1.39–1.33 (m, 8 H, ^{3}CH_2, ^{4}CH_2); ^{13}C NMR (101 MHz, $CDCl_3$) δ 170.6, 170.6, 170.1, 169.9, 169.8, 169.7, 169.7, 165.9, 127.8, 129.0 (toluene), 128.2 (toluene), 127.6, 97.5, 69.7, 69.1, 68.4, 68.1, 66.2, 62.5, 48.0, 46.5, 29.6, 29.2, 27.7, 26.8, 26.7, 25.9, 25.9, 20.9, 20.7, 20.7, 20.7; IR (KBr, cm^{-1}): 2937 (C−H), 2862 (C−H), 1751 (C=O), 1647 (C=C), 1611 (C=O), 1433 (C−H), 1373 (C−H); MALDI-TOF-MS m/z: [M+Na]$^+$ Calcd for $C_{43}H_{65}N_1Na_1O_{21}^+$: 954.3941, found: 954.3948; [M+K]$^+$ Calcd for $C_{43}H_{65}K_1N_1O_{21}^+$: 970.3681, found: 970.3675.

Supplementary Materials: The following are available online. ^{1}H and ^{13}C NMR spectra of **2** and **3** (Figures S1 and S2), and MALDI-TOF-mass and FTIR spectra of **3** (Figures S3 and S4).

Author Contributions: Conceptualization, A.M. and H.Y.; Investigation, S.O. and A.M.; Writing—original draft preparation and review and editing, A.M. All authors have read and agreed to the published version of the manuscript.

Funding: This research received no external funding.

Institutional Review Board Statement: Not applicable.

Informed Consent Statement: Not applicable.

Data Availability Statement: The data presented in this study are available in this article and Supplementary Materials.

Conflicts of Interest: The authors declare no conflict of interest.

References

1. Ohtsubo, K.; Marth, J.D. Glycosylation in Cellular Mechanisms of Health and Disease. *Cell* **2006**, *126*, 855–867. [CrossRef] [PubMed]
2. Varki, A. Biological Roles of Glycans. *Glycobiology* **2017**, *27*, 3–49. [CrossRef] [PubMed]
3. Lakshminarayanan, A.; Richard, M.; Davis, B.G. Studying Glycobiology at the Single-Molecule Level. *Nat. Rev. Chem.* **2018**, *2*, 148–159. [CrossRef]

4. Cummings, R.D. Stuck on Sugars–How Carbohydrates Regulate Cell Adhesion, Recognition, and Signaling. *Glycoconj. J.* **2019**, *36*, 241–257. [CrossRef] [PubMed]
5. Becer, C.R. The Glycopolymer Code: Synthesis of Glycopolymers and Multivalent Carbohydrate–Lectin Interactions. *Macromol. Rapid Commun.* **2012**, *33*, 742–752. [CrossRef] [PubMed]
6. Miyagawa, A.; Kurosawa, H.; Watanabe, T.; Koyama, T.; Terunuma, D.; Matsuoka, K. Synthesis of Glycoconjugate Polymer Carrying Globotriaose as Artificial Multivalent Ligand for Shiga Toxin-Producing Escherichia Coli O157: H7. *Carbohydr. Polym.* **2004**, *57*, 441–450. [CrossRef]
7. Abdouni, Y.; Yilmaz, G.; Becer, C.R. Sequence and Architectural Control in Glycopolymer Synthesis. *Macromol. Rapid Commun.* **2017**, *38*, 1700212. [CrossRef] [PubMed]
8. Li, J.; Zacharek, S.; Chen, X.; Wang, J.; Zhang, W.; Janczuk, A.; Wang, P.G. Bacteria Targeted by Human Natural Antibodies Using α-Gal Conjugated Receptor-Specific Glycopolymers. *Bioorg. Med. Chem.* **1999**, *7*, 1549–1558. [CrossRef]
9. Miyagawa, A.; Kasuya, M.C.Z.; Hatanaka, K. Inhibitory Effects of Glycopolymers Having Globotriose and/or Lactose on Cytotoxicity of Shiga Toxin 1. *Carbohydr. Polym.* **2007**, *67*, 260–264. [CrossRef]
10. Serizawa, T.; Yasunaga, S.; Akashi, M. Synthesis and Lectin Recognition of Polystyrene Core−Glycopolymer Corona Nanospheres. *Biomacromolecules* **2001**, *2*, 469–475. [CrossRef]
11. Miura, Y.; Koketsu, D.; Kobayashi, K. Synthesis and Properties of a Well-Defined Glycopolymer via Living Radical Polymerization. *Polym. Adv. Technol.* **2007**, *18*, 647–651. [CrossRef]
12. Lee, S.-G.; Brown, J.M.; Rogers, C.J.; Matson, J.B.; Krishnamurthy, C.; Rawat, M.; Hsieh-Wilson, L.C. End-Functionalized Glycopolymers as Mimetics of Chondroitin Sulfate Proteoglycans. *Chem. Sci.* **2010**, *1*, 322–325. [CrossRef] [PubMed]
13. Miyagawa, A.; Yamamura, H. Synthesis of β-1,3-Glucan Mimics by β-1,3-Glucan Trisaccharyl Monomer Polymerization. *Carbohydr. Polym.* **2020**, *227*, 115105. [CrossRef] [PubMed]
14. Miyagawa, A.; Watanabe, M.; Igai, K.; Kasuya, M.C.Z.; Natori, Y.; Nishikawa, K.; Hatanaka, K. Development of Dialyzer with Immobilized Glycoconjugate Polymers for Removal of Shiga-Toxin. *Biomaterials* **2006**, *27*, 3304–3311. [CrossRef] [PubMed]
15. Kiessling, L.; Grim, L.C.; Glycopolymer, J. Probes of Signal Transduction. *Chem. Soc. Rev.* **2013**, *42*, 4476–4491. [CrossRef] [PubMed]
16. Ma, Z.; Zhu, X.X. Copolymers Containing Carbohydrates and Other Biomolecules: Design, Synthesis and Applications. *J. Mater. Chem. B* **2019**, *7*, 1361–1378. [CrossRef] [PubMed]
17. Pramudya, I.; Chung, H. Recent Progress of Glycopolymer Synthesis for Biomedical Applications. *Biomater. Sci.* **2019**, *7*, 4848–4872. [CrossRef] [PubMed]

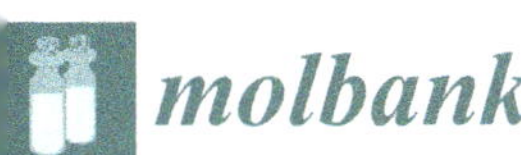

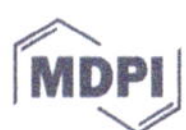

Short Note

Poly[3-methyl-1,3-oxazolidin-2-iminium[μ_3-cyanido-tri-μ_2-cyanido-κ^9C:N-tricuprate(I)]]

Leena N. Rachid and Peter W. R. Corfield *

Chemistry Department, Fordham University, 441 East Fordham Road, Bronx, New York, NY 10458, USA; lrachid@fordham.edu

* Correspondence: pcorfield@fordham.edu; Tel.: +1-718-817-4454

Abstract: The unexpected formation of an oxazole ring has occurred during synthesis of a copper(I) cyanide network polymer as part of our ongoing studies of the structural chemistry of these networks. Crystals of the title compound were formed during the synthesis of a previously reported CuCN network solid containing protonated *N*-methylethanolamine and have been characterized by single crystal X-ray structure analysis. The structure shows well-defined oxazole-2-iminium cations sitting in continuous channels along the short a-axis of the crystal in a new three-dimensional copper(I) cyanide polymeric network. Evidently, a reaction has occurred between the cyanide ion and the protonated *N*-methylethanolamine base.

Keywords: oxazole; iminium; unexpected product; copper cyanide; network; cuprophilic

Citation: Rachid, L.N.; Corfield, P.W.R. Poly[3-methyl-1,3-oxazolidin-2-iminium[μ_3-cyanido-tri-μ_2-cyanido-κ^9C:N-tricuprate(I)]]. *Molbank* **2021**, *2021*, M1259. https://doi.org/10.3390/M1259

Academic Editors: Stefano D'Errico and Annalisa Guaragna

Received: 15 June 2021
Accepted: 16 July 2021
Published: 26 July 2021

Publisher's Note: MDPI stays neutral with regard to jurisdictional claims in published maps and institutional affiliations.

1. Introduction

We report here the unexpected formation of poly[3-methyl-1,3-oxazolidin-2-iminium[μ_3-cyanido-tri-μ_2-cyanido-κ^9C:N-tricuprate(I)]], (**1**, Scheme 1) during preparative studies of NaCN/CuCN/*N*-methylethanolamine (meoen) mixtures as part of our ongoing studies of the structural chemistry of copper(I) cyanide networks. The usual product was [meoenH][$Cu_2(CN)_3$], **2**, (Scheme 1) obtained as tetragonal crystals after one or two weeks, with a structure that contains meoenH cations embedded in an anionic three-dimensional CuCN network [1]. In efforts to obtain more product, we allowed further fractions to crystallize from the filtrates. The title compound was obtained from such fractions as crystals with a platelike morphology rather than the rods usually obtained for the expected compound **2**. The crystal structure analysis reported here shows that a reaction between the cyanide ion and the ethanolamine cation has occurred (Scheme 2) to cause ring closure and the formation of an *N*-methylated 1,3-oxazole ring with a 2-iminium group, which acts as cation guest in a 3D anionic copper(I) cyanide network. Oxazole chemistry is a mature field [2–5] and oxazoles play an important role in pharmaceutical chemistry [6]. Oxazole synthesis has been achieved in at least fifteen different types of reactions [4], but we are not aware of a reaction similar to that reported here. There is less literature on the 2-iminium derivatives, and a search of the Cambridge Structural Database (CSD) [7] indicated only three crystallographic studies of their 2-iminium salts [8–10]. Reference 8 gives the structure of an oxaolidin-2-iminium ring with a seven-membered ring fused at C4 and C5, whereas the other references refer to the simple ring with various substituents.

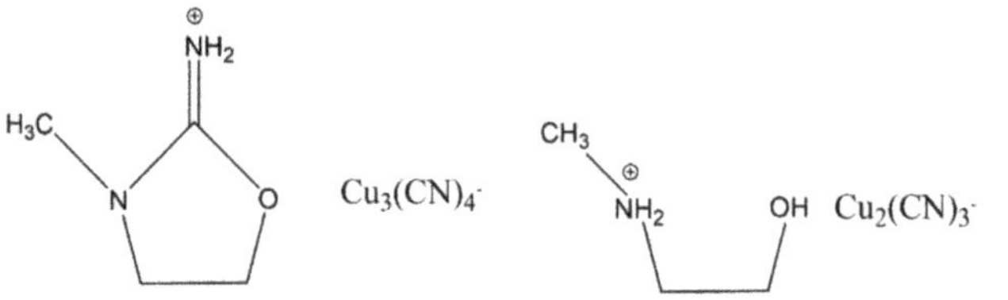

3-methyloxazolidin-2-iminium 2-hydroxy-*N*-methylethan-1-aminium (meoenH)

1 2

Scheme 1. Structures of the title compound, **1**, and of the expected product, **2**.

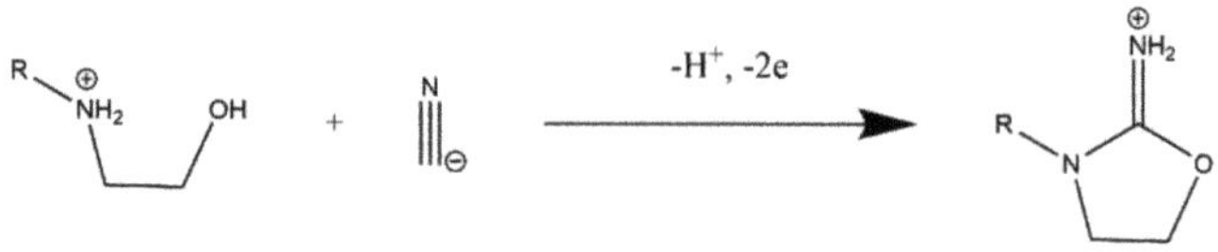

Scheme 2. Reaction of protonated N-methylethanolamine with cyanide ion.

2. Results

2.1. Synthesis

The title compound, **1**, is almost always obtained from the second or third crystal fraction from aqueous mixtures of the neutralized *N*-methylethanolamine and CuCN/NaCN solutions after two or more weeks. Inevitably the first fraction obtained contains crystals of **2**, sometimes mixed with a green powder. Although we have varied concentrations and the pH, we have not yet developed a procedure that will reliably give **1** as the first fraction. A typical synthesis involved mixing 0.90 g (10 mmol) of CuCN with 0.78 g (16 mmol) of NaCN in 60 mL of water until dissolved and adding a solution with volume 95 mL containing 3.00 g (40 mmol) meoen base neutralized with HCl(aq) to a pH of 2. The first precipitated fraction was filtered off after two weeks, and a second fraction filtered three weeks later gave 0.17 g of **1** as colorless plates, from which the crystal used for the X-ray analysis was selected. When air was excluded, no solid precipitated, suggesting that dioxygen from the air was the oxidant.

Sometimes pale or dark green crystals of **1** were obtained, shown by X-ray analysis to have the same structure as reported here. The dark green "crystals" shown in Figure 1 were very irregular in shape, yet diffracted well, and showed no extra diffraction pattern due to a separate phase. Examination optically at higher magnification (Figure S2) and with a scanning electron microscope (Figure S3) confirmed the presence of what looks like an amorphous phase deposited on crystalline material. Some of the sample was ground and examined by electron spin resonance—separate green and white particles were now visible. The esr spectrum, recorded as a first derivative absorption curve, (Figure S4) clearly shows the presence of Cu(II). Cu(II)-N bonding is indicated by the sharp secondary hyperfine lines that correspond the interaction of ^{14}N with the unpaired electron associated with the Cu(II) ion. We conclude that the "green" crystals are composed of colorless crystalline plates of **1** capped with deposits of a green amorphous phase that contains Cu(II), probably in the form of a mixed-valence copper cyanide complex. A similar phenomenon was reported in the analysis of the meoenH complex, **2** [1].

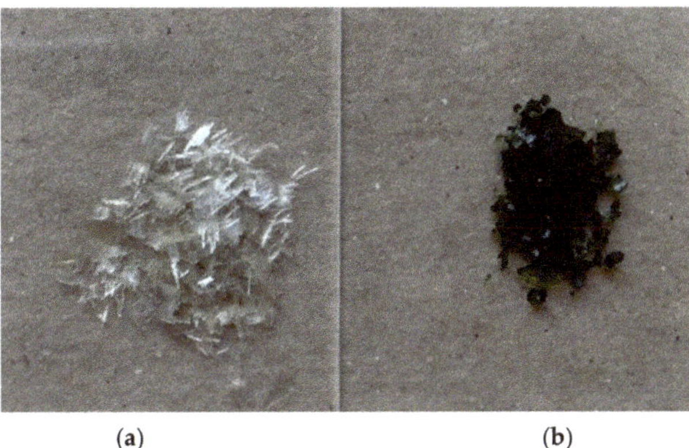

Figure 1. Photograph of crystalline samples of **1**. (**a**) Colorless plates; (**b**) plates coated with green amorphous material, as text describes.

2.2. X-Ray Structure

The crystal structure is built up from the oxazolidin-2-iminium cations in channels in a three-dimensional Cu(I)CN network with overall stoichiometry [LH][$Cu_3(CN)_4$], where LH represents the cation. Figure 2a presents the crystallographic asymmetric unit, showing the thermal ellipsoids and atom numbering. Figure 2b shows geometrical parameters for the oxazolidin-2-iminium cation. Atom numbering follows the typical convention for these rings; in the crystal structure, they are O11, C12, N13, C14, etc., to avoid confusion with the cyanide atom numbers. The bond distances around C2 are essentially equal at 1.30 Å, indicating resonance between three hybrid structures with the positive charge spread over O1, N3, and N7. The four atoms O1, C2, N3, N7 are strictly coplanar, but the constraints of the five-membered ring and its asymmetry force significant deviations from the idealized 120° angles: the internal angle is reduced to 114.1(3)°, while the external angle N7-C2-N3 at 127.2(4)° is much larger than the angle N7-C2-O1, at 118.8(4)°. A similar geometry for this portion of the cation is seen in the three X-ray structures of similar iminium cations mentioned earlier [8–10], even in reference [8], where there is no substituent on N3. Other bond lengths and angles seem normal.

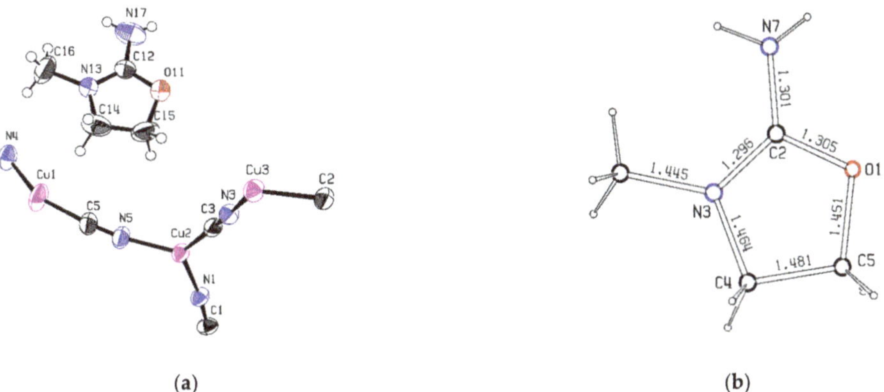

Figure 2. (**a**) Asymmetric unit for 1, showing thermal ellipsoids with 50% probability. Only one orientation of the disordered CN groups is shown. The CN groups C2≡N2 and C4≡N4 are each disordered about one of the inversion centers in the unit cell. (**b**) Bond lengths in the oxazolidin-2-iminium cation. Estimated standard deviations range from 0.004–0.007 Å.

Each of the three Cu atoms in the CuCN network is involved in a cuprophilic interaction, with Cu1 close to Cu2(x−1,y,z), and Cu3 close to Cu3(2−x,−y,1−z). Such weak d^{10}-d^{10} interactions are well known in Cu^{I} complexes, and have been explored in a recent review [11]. They are common in our CuCN network studies. Each Cu atom has a different geometry, as seen in Figure 3. Cu1 has a distorted digonal geometry, with average Cu-CN distance of 1.864(3) Å and angle at the Cu atom of 154.5(2)° and is 2.632(1) Å from Cu2(x−1,y,z). This cuprophilic interaction is without the bridging group(s) usually found in such structures, that help bring the Cu atoms close together—in the case of the CuCN structures, a μ_3 CN bridge. The present structure is unusual in this regard, as the cyanide group C3≡N3 clearly seems to act as a μ_2 bridging ligand, not as a μ_3 bridge. It could possibly be regarded as forming a very asymmetric μ_3 bridge, with C3-Cu1(1+x,y,z) and C3-Cu2 distances of 2.631(3) Å and 1.929(3) Å, but 2.631 Å is longer than any Cu-CN distances seen in a series of 63 μ_3CN-Cu_2 bridging bonds found in the Cambridge Structural Database [7], and the extreme asymmetry would lead one to expect a much greater Cu ... Cu distance than that found in the present structure [12]. Apart from its cuprophilic interaction with Cu1, atom Cu2 is trigonally coordinated with average Cu-CN distance of 1.934(3) Å and angles varying from 116.1(1)° to 125.6(1)°. Cu3 is in a rough tetrahedral coordination to cyanide groups, with also a close interaction with Cu3(2−x,−y,1−z), related by an inversion center. The Cu3 atoms are 2.730(1) Å apart and are bridged asymmetrically by a pair of symmetry related μ_3 C1≡N1 groups, with Cu-CN distances of 2.013(3) Å and 2.397(3) Å. The remaining two Cu-CN distances are shorter, with Cu3-N2 =1.938(3) Å and Cu3-N3 = 1.964(3) Å.

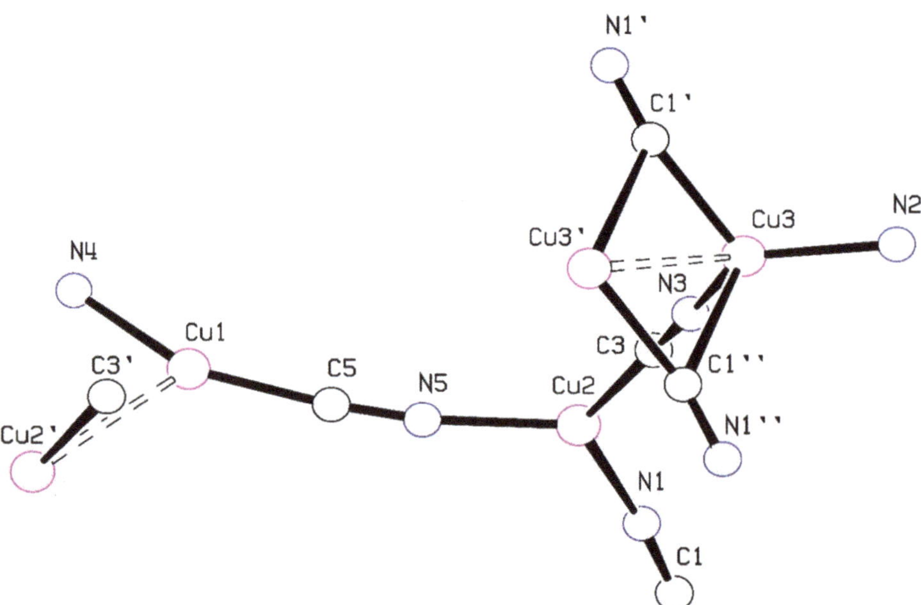

Figure 3. Coordination of the three copper atoms. Primed atoms are related by symmetry. Cuprophilic interactions are shown as dashed bonds.

The CuCN 3D network can be considered as made up of roughly planar networks connected by approximately vertical Cu-CN-Cu linkages which form walls to channels along the a-axis direction that contain the oxazalone-iminium cations, Figure 4. The planar networks are made up of 24-membered rings composed of repeated -Cu2-C3N3-Cu3-C1N1-Cu2-linkages with the Cu3 cuprophilic pairs acting as nodes where four rings meet. A

Cu1-C4≡N4-Cu1 group forms a belt across the center of each 24-membered ring via the cuprophilic Cu1 ... Cu2 interactions. As seen in Figure 4a, the cations pack neatly into channels in the CuCN network. There are no obvious H-bonding interactions between the cations and the anionic CuCN network.

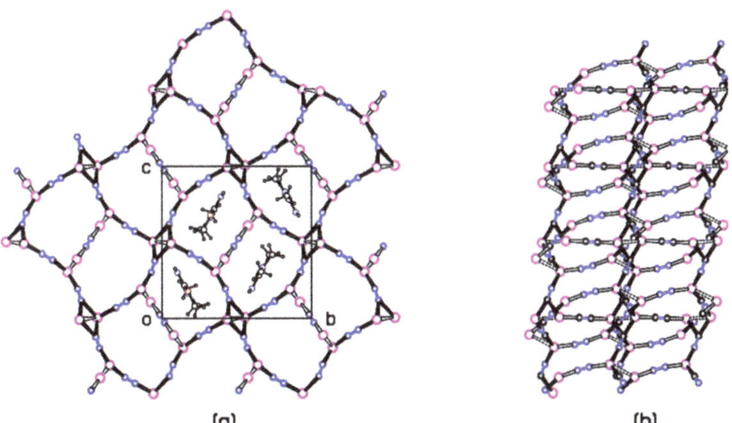

Figure 4. CuCN network and packing. (**a**) View down a-axis, showing the belted 24-membered rings. Oxazolidin cations shown only in the unit cell outline. (**b**) View down b-axis, showing the rings edge on linked by cyanide groups into the 3D structure. Cell outline is not included in this view. Magenta: Cu; red: O; blue: N; black: C or H.

2.3. Spectroscopy and Analyses

The infrared spectrum of **1** (Figure S5) shows strong absorptions due to C≡N stretching at 2082, 2106, and 2138 cm^{-1}. The absorption at 2106 cm^{-1} is probably due to μ_2 bridging CN groups 2, 3, and 5, as we see single absorptions close to this value in our CuCN structures that contain only this type of CN group [13,14] and other unpublished results]. The absorption at 2082 cm^{-1} will be due to the μ_3 bridging CN group as in Reference 1. The absorption at the higher energy, 2138 cm^{-1}, is likely due to C4≡N4, which bridges two digonal low-coordinate Cu1 atoms.

Strong absorptions due to the iminium N-H bonds occur at 3357 and 3461 cm^{-1} which may be compared with the absorptions at 3406 and 3497 cm^{-1} seen in the guanidinium cation in a CuCN network [14]. There are two other weak bands at 3182 and 3290 cm^{-1}. Other features of the ir spectrum include very strong absorbances at 1303, 1519, 1596, and 1705 cm^{-1}.

The elemental analysis of **1** gave 24.36%C, 2.12%H and 21.16%N, which are comparable with the values calculated for the new product, 24.27%C, 2.29%H and 21.24%N. The %Cu of 46.55% found was somewhat lower than the expected value of 48.16%.

3. Experimental Section

Crystal data for $C_8H_9Cu_3N_6O$ (M = 395.84 g/mol): crystal was a plate with dimensions 0.36 × 0.20 × 0.09 mm, monoclinic, space group $P2_1/c$ (no. 14), a = 6.9393(1) Å, b = 13.4468(3) Å, c = 13.4972(3) Å, β = 95.071(1)°, V = 1254.55(4) $Å^3$, Z = 4, T = 300(2) K, μ(MoKα) = 5.03 mm^{-1}, Dcalc = 2.096 g/cm^3, Dmeas = 2.08(1) g/cm^3, 19,265 reflections measured ($1.0° \leq \Theta \leq 27.48°$, 2867 unique (Rint = 0.046), which were used in all calculations. The final R_1 was 0.0344 ($I > 2\sigma(I)$) and wR_2 was 0.0790 (all data) for 175 variables. The structure was solved by the heavy atom method from a Patterson map calculated with SHELXS and refined with SHELXL Version 2017 [15]. All CN groups were modeled with disorder in their orientation. CN groups 2 and 4 were given 50% C/N occupancies, as they bridged an inversion center, and CN group 1 because the refined occupancies did not differ significantly from 50%. Occupancies for the major orientation for disordered CN groups 3 and 5 refined to 81(3)% and 78(4)%, respectively. Hydrogen atoms on C were constrained at idealized positions, riding on the carbon atoms, with C–H distances of 0.96 Å for methyl groups and 0.97 Å for methylene groups, and isotropic temperature factors 50% larger than the Ueq of the bonded C atoms. The iminium H atoms were refined independently with only a minimum restraint on distance. The cif file for this structure is included in the Supplementary Materials for this article and has also been deposited with the Cambridge Crystallographic Data Center as CCDC 2088682. These data can be obtained free of charge via http://www.ccdc.cam.ac.uk/conts/retrieving.html (accessed date: 15 June 2021) or from the CCDC, 12 Union Road, Cambridge CB2 1EZ, UK; Fax: +44 1223 336033; E-mail deposit@ccdc.cam.ac.uk).

4. Discussion

This work has shown the formation of a 3-methyl-1,3-oxazolidin-2-iminium cation via the reaction of a cyanide ion and protonated *N*-methylethanolamine in aqueous solution in the presence of CuCN/NaCN. In ongoing work on this system, we are attempting to find reaction conditions and pH levels that favor the formation of the title compound, to isolate salts of the cation that are independent of the copper cyanide network, and to develop an understanding of the reaction mechanism.

5. Materials and Methods

Chemicals were used as obtained from suppliers without further purification. The X-ray structure was determined with diffraction data collected with a Nonius Kappa CCD system (Bruker Axis LLC, Madison, WI, USA) using graphite monochromated MoKα radiation with $\lambda = 0.7107$ Å. Chemical analysis was performed by Robertson Microlit (Ledgewood, NJ, USA). FTIR data were obtained with a Nicolet iS50 FT-IR spectrometer (Thermo Fisher Scientific, Waltham, MA, USA. The SEM image was collected with a Zeiss Evo MA10 Scanning Electron Microscope and the esr spectrum was obtained with a Bruker EMXNano spectrometer.

Supplementary Materials: Figure S1: Checkcif Report, Figure S2: Optical photo of green "crystal" at high magnification; Figure S3: SEM picture of a different green "crystal"; Figure S4: esr spectrum of green sample; Figure S5: Infrared spectrum of title compound. MOL File, cif file.

Author Contributions: P.W.R.C. designed the experiments, carried out the X-ray analysis, analyzed the results and wrote the manuscript. L.N.R. carried out the syntheses and ir spectra. All authors have read and agreed to the published version of the manuscript.

Funding: This research received no external funding.

Institutional Review Board Statement: Not Applicable.

Informed Consent Statement: Not Applicable.

Data Availability Statement: The data presented in this study are available on request from the corresponding author.

Acknowledgments: We gratefully acknowledge support from the chemistry department at Fordham University, and we thank colleagues C. Koenigsmann for assistance with the electron microscopy and C. Bender for the esr measurements. Students A. Felix Varona, T. DaCunha and N. Eisha assisted with follow-up syntheses and density measurements.

Conflicts of Interest: The authors declare no conflict of interest.

References

1. Koenigsmann, C.; Rachid, L.N.; Sheedy, C.M.; Corfield, P.W.R. Synthesis, decomposition studies and crystal structure of a three-dimensional CuCN network structure with protonated N-methylethanolamine as the guest cation. *Acta Crystallogr. Sect. C Struct. Chem.* **2020**, *76*, 405–411. [CrossRef] [PubMed]
2. Wiley, R.H. The chemistry of the oxazoles. *Chem. Rev.* **1945**, *37*, 389–437. [CrossRef] [PubMed]

3. Lakhan, R.; Ternai, B. Advances in oxazole chemistry. *Adv. Heterocycl. Chem.* **1974**, *17*, 99–211.
4. Turchi, I.J.; Dewar, M.J.S. The Chemistry of Oxazoles. *Chem. Rev.* **1975**, *75*, 401–442. [CrossRef]
5. Turchi, I.J. Oxazole chemistry: A review of recent advances. *Ind. Eng. Chem. Prod. Res. Dev.* **1981**, *20*, 32–76. [CrossRef]
6. Kakkar, S.; Narasimhan, B. A comprehensive review on biological activities of oxazole derivatives. *BMC Chem.* **2019**, *13*, 16. [CrossRef] [PubMed]
7. Groom, C.R.; Bruno, I.J.; Lightfoot, M.P.; Ward, S.C. The Cambridge Structural Database. *Acta Cryst. B* **2016**, *72*, 317–325. [CrossRef] [PubMed]
8. Rynearson, K.D.; Dutta, S.; Tran, K.; Dibrov, S.M.; Hermann, T. Synthesis of Oxazole Analogs of Streptolidine Lactam. *Eur. J. Org. Chem.* **2013**, *2013*, 7337–7342. [CrossRef]
9. Cruz, A.; Padilla-Martínez, I.I.; García-Báez, E.V.; Contreras, R. Reactivity of Chlorodeoxypseudoephedrines with Oxo-, Thio-, and Selenocyanates. *Tetrahedron Asymmetry* **2007**, *18*, 123–130. [CrossRef]
10. Misaiszek, C.; Jarry, C.; Ouhabi, J.; Carpy, Y. Synthesis and Structural Study of 3-(2-propanone) 5-phenoxymethyl 2-iminooxazolidine: C13H16N2O3HCl. *Comptes Rendue L'Academie Sci. Ser. II* **1988**, *307*, 1189–1193.
11. Satyachand Harisomayajula, N.V.; Makovetskyi, S.; Tsai, Y.-C. Cuprophilic Interactions in and between Molecular Entities. *Chem. Eur. J.* **2019**, *25*, 8936–8954. [CrossRef] [PubMed]
12. Stocker, F.B.; Staeva, T.P.; Rienstra, C.M.; Britton, D. Crystal Structures of a Series of Complexes Produced by Reactions of Copper(I) Cyanide with Diamines. *Inorg. Chem.* **1999**, *38*, 984–991. [CrossRef]
13. Corfield, P.W.R.; Stavola, T.J. Poly[diethylammonium [tetra-μ_2-cyanido-κ^8C:*N*-tricuprate(I)]], a two-dimensional network solid. *IUCrData* **2020**, *5*, x200968. [CrossRef]
14. Corfield, P.W.R.; Dayrit, J.R. Poly[1,3-Dimethyltetrahydropyrimidin-2(1H)-iminium [tri-μ_2-cyanido-κ^6C:N-dicuprate(I)]]. *Molbank* **2020**, *4*, M1170. [CrossRef]
15. Sheldrick, G.M. Crystal structure refinement with SHELXL. *Acta Crystallogr. Sect. C Struct. Chem.* **2015**, *71*, 3–8. [CrossRef]

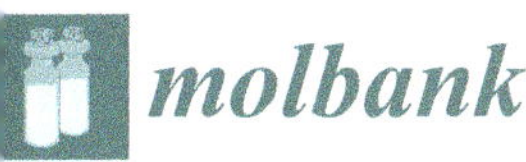

molbank

MDPI

Short Note

3-Isobutyl-5,5,7-tris(3-methylbut-2-en-1-yl)-1-phenyl-1,7-dihydro-4*H*-indazole-4,6(5*H*)-dione

José Edmilson Ribeiro do Nascimento, Daniela Hartwig, Raquel Guimarães Jacob * and Márcio Santos Silva *

Laboratório de Síntese Orgânica Limpa–LASOL, CCQFA, Universidade Federal de Pelotas–UFPel, P.O. Box 354, Pelotas 96010-900, RS, Brazil; jedmilsonrn@gmail.com (J.E.R.d.N.); dani.hartwig@gmail.com (D.H.)

* Correspondence: raquel.jacob@ufpel.edu.br (R.G.J.); silva.ms@ufpel.edu.br (M.S.S.)

Abstract: Here we describe the functionalization of lupulone natural compound in obtaining 3-Isobutyl-5,5,7-tris(3-methylbut-2-en-1-yl)-1-phenyl-1,7-dihydro-4*H*-indazole-4,6(5*H*)-dione. The lupulone-*H*-indazole derivative was prepared with 75% yield through the reaction between lupulone and phenyl-hydrazine employing $SiO_2/ZnCl_2$ (30% m/m) as a support solid in a solvent-free condition. Based on the possibilities of products, a complete NMR structural characterization of this lupulone-*H*-indazole was performed by ^1H, $^{13}C\{^1H\}$, COSY, HSQC and HMBC NMR experiments, showing an important contribution in producing the first results related to lupulone reactivity.

Keywords: soft resin; lupulone-indazole; NMR Spectroscopy; solvent-free

Citation: Nascimento, J.E.R.d.; Hartwig, D.; Jacob, R.G.; Silva, M.S. 3-Isobutyl-5,5,7-tris(3-methylbut-2-en-1-yl)-1-phenyl-1,7-dihydro-4*H*-indazole-4,6(5*H*)-dione. *Molbank* **2022**, *2022*, M1330. https://doi.org/10.3390/M1330

Academic Editors: Stefano D'Errico and Annalisa Guaragna

Received: 29 December 2021
Accepted: 29 January 2022
Published: 1 February 2022

1. Introduction

Biomass is renewable organic material that comes from animals and plants [1]. These materials are getting the attention of researchers due to the chemical transformation ability, which can lead to molecules with therapeutic potential or great industrial applicability [1,2].

Humulus lupulus L. has long been used as a medicinal plant, and its benefits include blood purification, treatment of inflammation, and sedative properties [3]. The compounds present in the extracts or essential oil of this plant have also been explored regarding their synthetic potential [4].

Hop is a base material in the brewing process to provide flavor and aroma to beer. Hop essential oil is present in the glandular cells of the hop plant, *Humulus lupulus* (Cannabinaceae) [5]. Among the vast number of natural compounds in the hop extract [6] are humulone and lupulone (Figure 1), which exhibit biological activity against some human cancer cells and have antibiofilm properties [7,8].

Figure 1. Structures of (−)-humulone and lupulone.

Based on our interest in the evaluation of the pharmacological properties of natural products [9,10], especially structural modification [11–14], we isolated lupulone from the hop plant. In this sense, the derivation of lupulone containing heterocyclic nitrogen represents a consolidated strategy to improve the pharmacological properties [11].

On the basis of these recent findings, we report here the first results related to the derivatization of lupulone through reaction with phenyl-hydrazine. Considering the lupulone structure and the possibilities of products, a full structural characterization was performed, which confirmed the formation of a *H*-indazole ring through ^{1}H, ^{13}C{^{1}H}, COSY HSQC, and HMBC NMR experiments.

2. Results and Discussion

Lupulone was isolated from soft resin fraction of hops in a 3% (m/m) yield after extraction and chromatographic purification, according to Taniguchi's method [15,16] The 3-Isobutyl-5,5,7-tris(3-methylbut-2-en-1-yl)-1-phenyl-1,7-dihydro-4*H*-indazole-4,6(5*H*) dione was obtained through a solvent-free reaction under conventional heating between lupulone and phenyl-hydrazine, in the presence of $SiO_2/ZnCl_2$ (30% m/m) solid support [17]. After chromatographic purification of the crude, the lupulone derivative **4** was isolated in a moderate yield (75%). The structure of the lupulone derivative **4** was supported by 1D and 2D NMR experiments and HRMS analysis, as can be seen in the characterization data (Section 3: Materials and Methods).

Initially, the reaction between lupulone and phenyl-hydrazine was optimized. As seen in Table 1, the presence of an acid support solid was essential to produce the lupulone derivative, as the presence of the reagents only was not sufficient to detect a product. The heating of the reaction media increased the yield, with the use of 60 °C demonstrating the best performance (Table 1, entry 5). When an excess of phenyl-hydrazine was employed the yield increased to 75% (Table 1, entry 6), although continuing to increase the amount of the phenyl-hydrazine did not enhance the reaction efficiency (Table 1, entry 6). The product highlighted in the Table 1 is the expected product in this functionalization.

Table 1. Optimization of the reaction between lupulone and phenyl-hydrazine.

Entry	Catalyst (56 mol %)	Lupulone: Hydrazine Ratio (mmol)	Temp. (°C)	Yield (%) [a]
1	–	(0.5:0.5)	60	–
2	$SiO_2/ZnCl_2$	(0.5:0.5)	60	51
3	$SiO_2/ZnCl_2$	(0.5:0.5)	25	20
4	$SiO_2/ZnCl_2$	(0.5:0.5)	100	31
5	$SiO_2/ZnCl_2$	(0.5:0.6)	60	75
6	$SiO_2/ZnCl_2$	(0.5:0.7)	60	76

[a] Yield of the isolated product.

At this moment, the main product was isolated by column chromatography; however several small by-products were also detected by thin-layer-chromatography of the crude reaction. Evaluation using mass spectrometry showed it was not possible to discriminate the product possibilities, because of mass similarities and the tautomerism effect (Figure 2). Additionally, when employing ^{1}H and ^{13}C{^{1}H} NMR experiments, it was possible to eliminate the lupulone derivatives **1**, **2**, and **5** (Figure 2), due the amount of aliphatic carbons, but this was not sufficient to clarify the lupulone derivatives **3**, **4** and **6** (see Figure 2). Thus, a full assignment was performed, for which 2D NMR experiments were also necessary. Based on this structural elucidation, COSY, HSQC and HMBC NMR experiments were carried out, and the NMR data were interpreted according to the Table 2

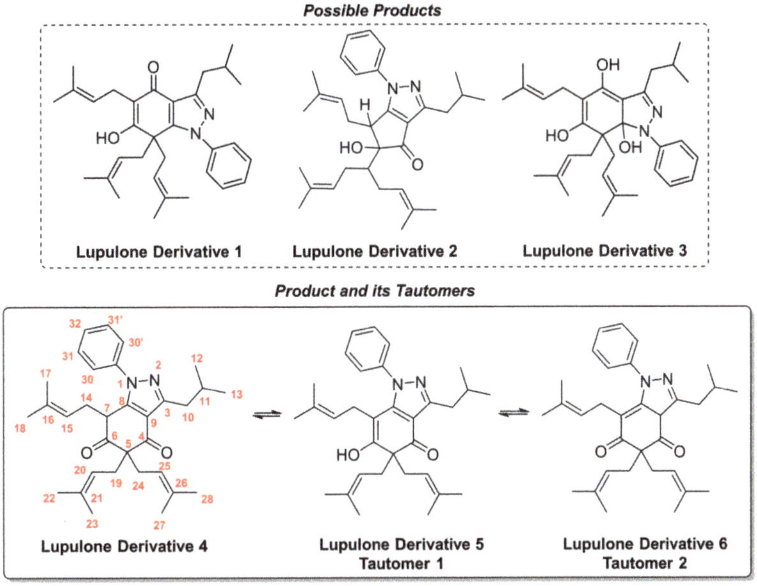

Figure 2. Possible products and full structural assignment of the lupulone derivative **4**.

Table 2. ^{1}H and ^{13}C chemical shifts, coupling constants, and HMBC 2D correlations of lupulone derivative **4**.

Number	^{1}H (ppm)	^{13}C (ppm)	^{1}H-^{13}C HMBC
1	—	—	—
2	—	—	—
3	—	153.6	—
4	—	193.1	—
5	—	65.7	—
6	—	210.0	—
7	3.89 (*dd*, *J* = 5.0 and 6.3 Hz)	46.8	6, 8, 9 and 14
8	—	147.1	—
9	—	118.6	—
10	2.98 (*d*, *J* = 7.2 Hz)	36.3	3 and 9
11	2.25 (*n*, *J* = 6.7 Hz)	28.1	3, 10, 12 and 13
12	1.07 (*d*, *J* = 6.7 Hz)	22.4	10 and 11
13	1.06 (*d*, *J* = 6.7 Hz)	22.3	10 and 11
14	2.10 (*ddd*, *J* = 6.3, 6.6 and 14.7 Hz)	30.1	6, 7, 8, 15 and 16
14′	2.55–2.70 (*m*)	30.1	6, 7, 8, 15 and 16
15	4.60 (*t*, *J* = 7.3 Hz)	118.4	14, 17 and 18
16	—	135.6	—
17	1.26 (s)	25.7	15 and 16
18	1.53 (s)	17.4	15 and 16
19	2.78 (*d*, *J* = 7.4 Hz)	33.9	4, 5, 6, 20 and 21
20	4.93 (*t*, *J* = 7.4 Hz)	118.1	19, 22 and 23
21	—	134.4	—
22	1.66 (*s*)	26.0	19, 20 and 21
23	1.72 (*s*)	18.0	19, 20 and 21
24	2.55–2.70 (*m*)	39.5	4, 5, 6, 25 and 26
25	4.94 (*t*, *J* = 7.3 Hz)	118.6	24, 27 and 28
26	—	135.1	—
27	1.53 (*s*)	25.9	24, 25 and 26

Table 2. *Cont.*

Number	^{1}H (ppm)	^{13}C (ppm)	^{1}H-^{13}C HMBC
28	1.67 (*s*)	17.7	24, 25 and 26
29	—	139.2	—
30	7.48–7.50 (*m*)	124.6	29 and 32
31	7.57–7.59 (*m*)	129.6	29
32	7.53–7.54 (*m*)	128.7	30

The 2D NMR experiments confirmed the formation of the *H*-indazole ring, according to the structural assignment (Figure 2). First, the ^{1}H spectrum (Figure S1) demonstrates a clear signal profile, with the aliphatic protons being easily identified (Table 2, methyl groups, numbers: 12, 13, 17, 18, 22, 23, 27 and 28), as well as the aromatic protons (Table 2, numbers 30, 31, 31′, 32). In a downfield ^{1}H chemical shift, it is possible to detect the vinylic signals (Table 2, numbers 15, 20 and 25) alongside an additional proton, established by integral values. This extra ^{1}H NMR signal in 3.9 ppm demonstrates a deshielded chemical shift due the proximity to nitrogen and carbonyl groups, or it could be derived from some hydroxyl group of the lupulone derivative **3** [18]. In a upfield region, it is possible to observe the aliphatic signals, considering the multiplicity standard (Table 2, numbers 10, 11, 14, 19 and 24). It is noteworthy that the protons 14 are diastereotopics with a distinct multiplicity profile (Table 2, numbers 14 and 14′, confirmed by HSQC), indicating the lupulone derivative **4** or its tautomer, with the lupulone derivative **6** as the possible product, due the presence of the aromatic ring near to these protons, which results in an anisotropic environment. Based on the COSY experiment, stronger correlations were observed between the protons 14 and 14′ with the deshielded aliphatic proton (number 7), which confirms the lupulone derivative **4** and excludes the lupulone derivative **6**.

According to the $^{13}C\{^{1}H\}$ spectrum (Figure S2), all 32 carbons can be visualized once no overlapping of signals occurred. The amount of aliphatic carbons corroborates with the *H*-indazole ring through the presence of an additional aliphatic carbon, differently from other probable products (Figure 2: lupulone derivatives **1**, **2** and **5**). Considering the aromatic region, only two downfield carbons are evident with a typical carbonyl chemical shift profile (Table 2, numbers 4 and 6, 193.0 and 209.9 ppm, respectively, confirmed by HMBC), which allows us to discard the lupulone derivative **3** due to the presence of phenol groups in the main structure [18]. Additionally, the *ortho* and *meta* carbons can be identified from aromatic ring based on the signal intensity. However, no further identifications could be evidenced without the HSQC and HMBC 2D NMR experiments (see NMR spectra in SI).

Although the ^{1}H and ^{13}C NMR profile can provide good evidence for the lupulone derivative **4** (Figure 2), more proof is necessary to confirm the main structure. Thus, a full structural elucidation is necessary to identify all protons and carbons signals, and for this purpose, 2D NMR experiments were carried out. As can be seen in Table 2, proton-carbon correlations are valuable for recognizing all NMR signals. Additionally, interpreting the COSY NMR experiment (Figure 3), the methyl groups 12 and 13 and the proton 10 were identified by the correlation with proton 11 (2.25 ppm, nonet) containing eight neighbor protons. In the same NMR region, the diastereotopic protons 14 and 14′ could be detected by the correlation between them and by a weak correlation with the vinylic proton 15, also confirming the methyl groups 17 and 18. The other two butene groups were recognized by the same correlation pattern, although no distinction among these groups was possible.

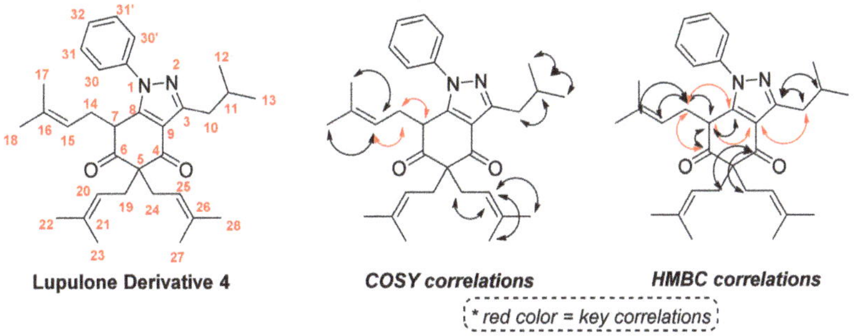

Figure 3. COSY and HMBC correlations in the lupulone derivative **4**.

Next, the HSQC NMR spectrum was evaluated (Figure S4). Based on the identification of the protons using proton–proton correlations, the carbons directly attached were detected. The aliphatic moiety was easily recognized, because there is only one quaternary carbon (Table 2, number 5). When the downfield region was checked, the vinylic carbons attached to the protons were identified (Table 2, numbers 15, 20 and 25) as were the *ortho*, *meta* and *para* carbons in the aromatic ring (Table 2, number 30, 31 and 32).

Finally, the HMBC NMR experiment was carried out to assign the quaternary carbons, confirming the main core of the lupulone derivative **4** (Figures S5–S7). In this way, to carry out the ^{1}H-^{13}C HMBC experiment, 10 Hz was used for the long-distance parameter (SI, CNST13), although this long-range term could be optimized for a proper assignment. Based on the proximity of protons and carbons, especially considering the stronger $^{3}J_{1H\text{-}13C}$ scalar coupling, the quaternary carbons were assigned. It is important to mention that the correlation between the diastereotopic protons 14 and 14′ and the carbons C6, C7, C8, C15 and C16 were also visualized in the HMBC NMR spectrum.

Analysis of HMBC NMR spectrum in the downfield region supports the formation of the lupulone derivative **4** (Figure 3). The quaternary carbon 3 was assigned by correlations with the protons 10 and 11, corroborating the typical ^{13}C chemical shift (Table 2; number 3; 153.6 ppm). The carbon 4 (carbonyl) can be confirmed by ^{3}J correlation with the protons 24 and 19 (Figure S7), but it does not have a correlation with the proton 7. The quaternary carbon-5 does not demonstrate correlation with the proton 7, which supports the lupulone derivative **4**. The carbon 6 demonstrates a similar profile with the ^{3}J correlation with the protons 7, 19 and 24. When we evaluated the carbon 7, only weak correlations were observed with the diastereotopic protons 14 and 14′. The carbon 8 was clearly assigned by the correlation with the proton 7 and a weak correlation with the diastereotopic protons 14 and 14′ (Figure S6). Finally, the carbon 9 was assigned by the correlations with the protons 7 and 10 (Figure 3).

The NMR experimental data completely support the lupulone derivative **4**. Although the possible tautomers of lupulone derivative **4** (Figure 2; tautomers 1 and 2) can change the chemical shift profile, their structures were not detected in the NMR spectra. Thus, to improve the discussion regarding the reactivity of the lupulone starting material, we propose a plausible mechanism (Figure 4) [19]. Initially, a keto-enol tautomerism justifies the formation of an aliphatic carbon in the main structure. The first step is the formation of imine from the reaction between ketone and amine organic functions, eliminating a water molecule. Afterward, a cyclization is favored, derived from the proximity between carbonyl and amine groups, followed by the elimination of the hydroxyl group (E1cB type). Finally, the base present in the media provides the formation of another carbonyl group, establishing the *H*-indazole ring and producing another water molecule. The formation of a heteroaromatic ring by the tautomerism effect affords the product lupulone derivative **4**, probably derived from the stability gain by the aromaticity (Figure 4). In addition, the lupulone derivative **2** was not observed; however, the ring contraction is a possible pathway, derived from an isomerization process [20]. Based on this mechanism, it is possible to visualize the formation of various other products derived from the different pathways in this reaction (Figure S8, lupulone derivatives **1** and **3**), justifying the need to perform a full structural assignment, as varying the reaction conditions could produce distinct products.

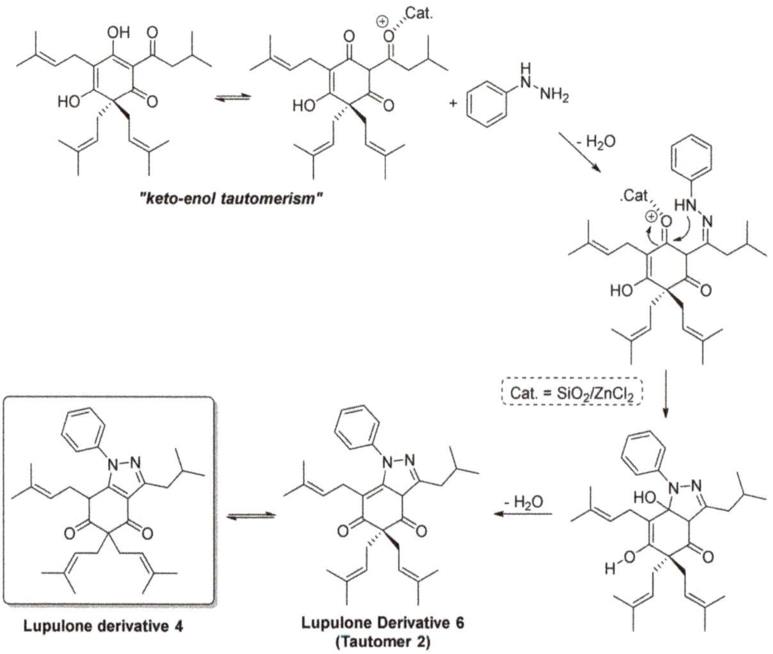

Figure 4. A plausible mechanism to obtain the lupulone derivative **4**.

3. Materials and Methods

The reactions were monitored by TLC carried out on pre-coated TLC sheets ALUGRAM® Xtra SIL G/UV_{254} by using UV light as the visualization agent and the mixture of 5% vanillin in 10% H_2SO_4 under heating conditions as the developing agent. Silica gel (particle size 63–200 μm) was used for flash chromatography. The reagents, solvents and chromatographic materials were purchased from Sigma-Aldrich® Brazil. The nuclear magnetic resonance (NMR) data were collected on a Bruker Avance III HD spectrometer (Bruker®, Atibaia, Brazil) operating at 400.0 MHz for ^1H and 100 MHz for ^{13}C. NMR data were recorded at 25 °C, with chemical shifts δ reported in parts per million and coupling constants J in Hertz. The NMR sample was prepared employing 5 mg of the respective lupulone derivative **4** in 600 μL deuterated chloroform. Chemical shifts of ^1H and $^{13}C\{^1H\}$ NMR experiments were referenced by TMS (tetramethylsilane) at δ = 0.0 ppm. Two-dimensional NMR experiments COSY, HSQC, and HMBC were performed using the standard Bruker pulse sequence with gradient. The relaxation delay, 90° pulse, spectral width, and number of data points for ^1H NMR were 1 s, 9.43 μs, 5580 Hz, and 64 K, respectively. The corresponding parameters for the ^{13}C NMR experiments were 0.5 s, 10.0 μs, 26,041 Hz, and 64 K, respectively. Two-dimensional experiments, including COSY, HSQC, and HMBC, were performed with 4 K × 512 ($t2 \times t1$) data points. The long-range coupling time for ^1H-^{13}C HMBC was 10 Hz. All data were analyzed using Bruker software (Topspin 3.6, Bruker®, Atibaia, Brazil). Low-resolution mass spectra (MS) were obtained with a Shimadzu GC-MS-QP2010 mass spectrometer (São Paulo, Brazil). The HRMS analyses were performed in a Bruker micrOTOF-QII spectrometer equipped with an APCI source operating in positive mode. The samples were solubilized in acetonitrile and analyzed by direct infusion at a constant flow rate of 180 μL/min. The acquisition parameters were capillary: 4000 V, end plate offset

−500 V, nebulizer: 1.5 bar, dry gas: 1.5 L min^{-1}, and dry heater: 180 °C. The collision cell energy was set to 5.0 eV. The mass-to-charge ratio (m/z) data were processed and analyzed using Bruker Daltonics software: Compass Data Analysis and Isotope Pattern.

Experimental Procedure to obtain the Lupulone Derivative **4**: The 3-Isobutyl-5,5,7-tris(3-methylbut-2-en-1-yl)-1-phenyl-1,7-dihydro-4*H*-indazole-4,6(5*H*)-dione was obtained through the reaction between lupulone (0.5 mmol) and phenyl-hydrazine (0.6 mmol) employing 20 mg (0.277 mmol) of $SiO_2/ZnCl_2$ (30% m/m) [17] as a support solid in a solvent-free condition. The reaction media was heated to 60 °C for 20 h. The conventional heating was removed and the heterogenous catalyst was filtred using a small amount of ethyl acetate (2.0 mL). Then, the solvent was removed without an extraction step, and the sample obtained was directly purified by column chromatography. The lupulone derivative **4** was isolated in a moderate yield (75%) by column chromatography, employing a mixture of *n*-hexane/ethyl acetate in a 94:04 ratio. The product is a yellow oil with a pleasant smell.

Lupulone Derivative **4** Characterization: Yield 75%, yellow oil. NMR ^1H ($CDCl_3$, 400 MHz) δ 0.98 (d, J = 3.0 Hz, 3H), 0.99 (d, J = 3.0 Hz, 3H), 1.18 (s, 3H), 1.44 (s, 3H), 1.53 (s, 3H); 1.57 (m, 6H); 1.63 (s, 3H); 2.10 (*ddd*, J = 6.3, 6.6 and 14.7 Hz), 2.13–2.18 (m, 1H), 2.50–2.60 (m, 3H), 2.70 (d, J = 7.3 Hz, 2H), 2.90 (d, J = 7.2 Hz, 2H), 3.84–3.79 (m, 1H), 4.51 (t, J = 7.2 Hz, 1H), 4.86 (t, J = 7.3 Hz, 2H), 7.47–7.37 (m, 3H), 7.55–7.47 (m, 2H). ^{13}C NMR (100 MHz, $CDCl_3$) δ 17.36; 17.69; 17.96; 22.34; 22.40; 25.71; 25.90; 25.93; 28.07; 30.11; 33.83; 36.32; 39.50; 46.74; 65.65; 118.12; 118.39; 118.58; 119.72; 124.54; 128.70; 129.59; 134.37; 135.05; 135.61; 139.21; 147.14; 153.56; 193.04; 209.92. MS (relative intensity) m/z: 486 (3); 417(39); 349(100); 333(15); 295(4); 251(2); 207(4); 77(5); 69(26); 41(29). IR (cm^{-1}): 3224, 2988, 2220, 1615, 1463, 942, 962, 784. HRMS (ESI): m/z $[M + H]^+$ calcd for $C_{32}H_{43}N_2O_2$: 487.33191; found: 487.33183.

4. Conclusions

In conclusion, we synthesized 3-Isobutyl-5,5,7-tris(3-methylbut-2-en-1-yl)-1-phenyl-1,7-dihydro-4*H*-indazole-4,6(5*H*)-dione and performed a full structural elucidation of its ^1H and $^{13}C\{^1H\}$ NMR signals. This is an important contribution to produce the first results related to lupulone reactivity, which could be used for pharmacological applications. Considering the lupulone derivative **4** accessed, these results highlight the possibilities for new derivatizations, especially considering the tautomerism effect.

Supplementary Materials: The following are available online. Figures S1–S7: ^1H, ^{13}C, COSY, HSQC and HMBC spectra, Figure S8. Mechanism to access the Lupulone Derivative **1** (Expected) and Lupulone Derivative **3** (not favored).

Author Contributions: R.G.J. supervised; M.S.S. designed and conceived the experiments and wrote, reviewed and edited the manuscript; D.H. wrote, reviewed and edited the manuscript; J.E.R.d.N. developed the synthetic methodology and performed the experiments. All authors have read and agreed to the published version of the manuscript.

Funding: This research was funded by CNPq (Grants 409782/2018-1, 308015/2019-3 and 309013/2019-4) and FAPERGS (ARD 19/2551-0001258-6) and partially financed by the Coordenação de Aperfeiçoamento de Pessoal de Nivel Superior-Brasil (CAPES), Finance Code 001.

Data Availability Statement: The data presented in this study are available in the Supplementary Materials for this article.

Acknowledgments: The authors are grateful to UFPel for providing support to carry out this work and the funding agencies for the financial support. Additionally, we would like to thank the reviewers for their revisions and comments, which were useful to understand the product obtained.

Conflicts of Interest: The authors declare no conflict of interest.

References

1. Jacob, R.G.; Oliveira, D.H.; Dias, I.F.C.; Schumacher, R.F.; Savegnago, L. Óleos essenciais como matéria-prima sustentável para o preparo de produtos com maior valor agregado. *Rev. Virtual Quim.* **2016**, *9*, 294–316. [CrossRef]
2. Gallezot, P. Conversion of biomass to selected Chemical products. *Chem. Soc. Rev.* **2012**, *41*, 1538–1558. [CrossRef] [PubMed]
3. Schultz, C.; Chiheb, C.; Pischetsrieder, M. Quantification os co-, n-, and ad-lupulone in hop-based dietary supplements and phytopharmaceuticals and modulation of their contentes by the extraction method. *J. Pharm. Biomed. Anal.* **2019**, *168*, 124–132. [CrossRef] [PubMed]
4. Tyrrell, E.; Archer, R.; Tucknott, M.; Colston, K.; Pirianov, G.; Ramanthan, D.; Dhillon, R.; Sinclair, A.; Skinner, G.A. The synthesis and anticancer effects of a range of natural and unnatural hop β-accids on breast câncer cells. *Phytochem. Lett.* **2012**, *5*, 144–149. [CrossRef]
5. Goese, M.; Kammhuber, K.; Bacher, A.; Zenk, M.H.; Eisenreich, W. Biosynthesis of bitter acids in hops. A ^{13}C-NMR and ^{2}H-NMR study on the building blocks of humulone. *Eur. J. Biochem.* **1999**, *263*, 447–454. [CrossRef] [PubMed]
6. Intelmann, D.; Haseleu, G.; Hofmann, T. LC-MS/MS Quantification of Hop-Derived Bitter Compounds in Beer Using the ECHO Technique. *J. Agric. Food Chem.* **2009**, *57*, 1172–1182. [CrossRef] [PubMed]
7. Tyrrel, E.; Archer, R.; Skinner, G.A.; Singh, K.; Colston, K.; Driver, C. Structure elucidation and an investigation into in vitro effects of hop acids on human cancer cells. *Phytochem. Lett.* **2010**, *3*, 17–23. [CrossRef]
8. Bogdanova, K.; Roderova, M.; Kolar, M.; Langova, K.; Dusek, M.; Jost, P.; Kubelkova, K.; Bostik, P.; Olsovska, J. Antibiofilm activity of bioactive hop compounds humulone, lupulone and xanthohumol toward susceptible and resistant staphylococci. *Res. Microbiol.* **2018**, *169*, 127–134. [CrossRef] [PubMed]
9. Castro, M.R.; Victoria, F.N.; Oliveira, D.H.; Jacob, R.G.; Savegnago, L.; Alves, D. Essential oil of Psidium cattleianum leaves: Antioxidant and antifungal activity. *Pharm. Biol.* **2015**, *53*, 242–250. [CrossRef] [PubMed]
10. Fonseca, A.O.S.; Pereira, D.I.B.; Jacob, R.G.; Maia Filho, F.S.; Oliveira, D.H.; Maroneze, B.P.; Valente, J.S.S.; Osório, L.G.; Botton, S.A.; Meireles, M.C.A. In vitro susceptibility of Brazilian Pythium insidiosum isolates to essential oil of some Lamiaceae Family species. *Mycopathologia* **2015**, *179*, 253–258. [CrossRef] [PubMed]
11. Lenardão, E.J.; Bottesselle, G.V.; Azambuja, F.; Perin, G.; Jacob, R.G. Citronellal as key compounds in organic synthesis. *Tetrahedron* **2007**, *63*, 6671–6712. [CrossRef]
12. Montenegro, L.M.P.; Griep, J.B.; Tavares, F.C.; Oliveira, D.H.; Bianchini, D.; Jacob, R.G. Synthesis and characterization of imine-modified silicas obtained by the reaction of essential oil of *Eucalyptus citriodora*, 3-aminopropyltriethoxysilane and tetraethylorthosilicate. *Vib. Spectrosc.* **2013**, *68*, 272–278. [CrossRef]
13. Chagas, A.C.; Domingues, L.F.; Fantatto, R.R.; Giglioti, R.; Oliveira, M.C.S.; Oliveira, D.H.; Mano, R.A.; Jacob, R.G. In vitro and in vivo acaricide action of juvenoid analogs produced from the chemical modification of *Cymbopogon* spp. and *Corymbia citriodora* essential oil on the cattle tick *Rhipicephalus* (Boophilus) microplus. *Veterin. Parasit.* **2014**, *205*, 277–284. [CrossRef] [PubMed]
14. Ferraz, M.C.; Mano, R.A.; Oliveira, D.H.; Maia, D.S.V.; Silva, W.P.; Savegnago, L.; Lenardão, E.J.; Jacob, R.G. Synthesis, Antimicrobial, and Antioxidant Activities of Chalcogen-Containing Nitrone Derivatives from (*R*)-Citronellal. *Medicines* **2017**, *4*, 39. [CrossRef] [PubMed]
15. Taniguchi, Y.; Taniguchi, H.; Yamada, M.; Matsukura, Y.; Koizumi, H.; Furihata, K.; Shindo, K. Analysis of the components of hard resin in hops (*Humulus lupulus L.*) and structural elucidation of their transformation products formed during the brewing process. *J. Agric. Food Chem.* **2014**, *62*, 11602–11612. [CrossRef] [PubMed]
16. Olsovska, J.; Bostikova, V.; Dusek, M.; Jandovska, V.; Bogdanova, K.; Cermak, P.; Bostik, P.; Mikyska, A.; Kolar, M. *Humulus Lupulus* L. (Hops)—A valuable source of compounds with bioactive effects for future therapies. *Mil. Med. Sci. Lett.* **2016**, *85*, 19–31. [CrossRef]
17. Radatz, C.S.; Rodrigues, M.B.; Alves, D.; PERIN, G.; Lenardão, E.J.; Savegnago, L.; Jacob, R.G. Synthesis of 1-*H*-1,5-benzodiazepines derivatives using $SiO_2/ZnCl_2$. *Heteroat. Chem.* **2011**, *22*, 180–185. [CrossRef]
18. Pretsch, E.; Bühlman, P.; Badertscher, M. *Structure Determination of Organic Compounds, Tables of Spectral Data*, 5th ed.; Springer: Berlin/Heidelberg, Germany, 2020. [CrossRef]
19. Briggs, L.H.; Penfold, A.R.; Short, W.F. Leptospermone. Part I. *J. Chem. Soc.* **1938**, 1193–1195. [CrossRef]
20. Dybowski, M.P.; Typek, R.; Bernacik, K.; Dawidowicz, A.L. Isomerization of bitter acids during the brewing process. *Ann. Univesitatis Marie Curie-Sklodowska Lub.-Pol.* **2015**, *2*, 137–144. [CrossRef]

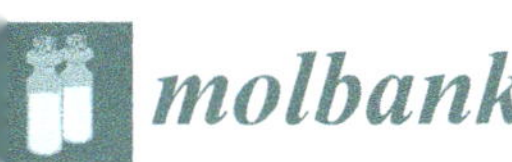 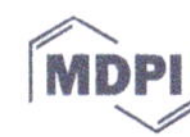

Short Note

O6-[(2″,3″-O-Isopropylidene-5″-O-^{t}butyldimethylsilyl)pentyl]-5′-O-^{t}butyldiphenylsilyl-2′,3′-O-isopropylideneinosine

Maria Marzano [1], Monica Terracciano [2], Vincenzo Piccialli [3], Ahmed Mahal [4,5,6], Roberto Nilo [7] and Stefano D'Errico [2,*]

1 Institute of Applied Sciences and Intelligent Systems (ISASI), Unity of Naples, National Research Council (CNR), via Campi Flegrei, 34, 80078 Naples, Italy; maria.marzano@na.isasi.cnr.it
2 Department of Pharmacy, University of Naples Federico II, via Domenico Montesano, 49, 80131 Naples, Italy; monica.terracciano@unina.it
3 Department of Chemical Sciences, University of Naples Federico II, via Cintia, 21, 80126 Naples, Italy; vinpicci@unina.it
4 Department of Medical Biochemical Analysis, College of Health Technology, Cihan University—Erbil, Erbil 44001, Kurdistan Region, Iraq; ahmed.mahal@cihanuniversity.edu.iq
5 Key Laboratory of Plant Resources Conservation and Sustainable Utilization, Guangdong Provincial Key Laboratory of Applied Botany, South China Botanical Garden, Chinese Academy of Sciences, Guangzhou 510650, China
6 Guangzhou HC Pharmaceutical Co., Ltd., Guangzhou 510663, China
7 Institute of Experimental Endocrinology and Oncology "Gaetano Salvatore" (IEOS) National Research Council (CNR), via T. De Amicis, 95, 80145 Naples, Italy; r.nilo@studenti.unina.it
* Correspondence: stefano.derrico@unina.it; Tel.: +39-081-679981

Abstract: Cyclic adenosine diphosphate ribose (cADPR) is a cyclic nucleotide involved in the Ca^{2+} homeostasis. In its structure, the northern ribose, bonded to adenosine through an N1 glycosidic bond, is connected to the southern ribose through a pyrophosphate bridge. Due to the chemical instability at the N1 glycosidic bond, new bioactive cADPR derivatives have been synthesized. One of the most interesting analogues is the cyclic inosine diphosphate ribose (cIDPR), in which the hypoxanthine replaced adenosine. The efforts for synthesizing new linear and cyclic northern ribose modified cIDPR analogues led us to study in detail the inosine N1 alkylation reaction. In the last few years, we have produced new flexible cIDPR analogues, where the northern ribose has been replaced by alkyl chains. With the aim to obtain the closest flexible cIDPR analogue, we have attached to the inosine N1 position a 2″,3″-dihydroxypentyl chain, possessing the two OH groups in a ribose-like fashion. The inosine alkylation reaction afforded also the O6-alkylated regioisomer, which could be a useful intermediate for the construction of new kinds of cADPR mimics.

Keywords: cADPR; nucleosides; nucleotides; inosine; alkylation; calcium mobilization; ryanodine receptor; primary cortical neurons

Citation: Marzano, M.; Terracciano, M.; Piccialli, V.; Mahal, A.; Nilo, R.; D'Errico, S. O6-[(2″,3″-O-Isopropylidene-5″-O-^{t}butyldimethylsilyl)pentyl]-5′-O-^{t}butyldiphenylsilyl-2′,3′-O-isopropylideneinosine. *Molbank* **2022**, *2022*, M1345. https://doi.org/10.3390/M1345

Academic Editor: Fawaz Aldabbagh

Received: 3 February 2022
Accepted: 23 February 2022
Published: 1 March 2022

1. Introduction

The design and synthesis of new nucleoside and nucleotide analogues is a frontier theme in light of the current SARS-CoV-2 pandemic that the world is facing [1]. However, apart from being employed in medicinal chemistry both as antiviral [2] and antitumor drugs [3], nucleosides, nucleotides, and their analogues can be also used as probes in the signaling pathways [4–6]. Cyclic nucleotides are important second messengers involved in signal transduction [7,8]. Among them, cADPR (**1**, Figure 1), an 18-membered cyclic nucleotide firstly isolated from sea urchin egg extracts [9], elicits Ca^{2+} ions from the endoplasmic reticulum (ER) to cytosol through the ryanodine receptor (RyR) in several cellular systems [10]. Alterations in the cADPR biosynthesis and calcium homeostasis can play pathological roles in diabetes, airway hyper-responsiveness and autism [11]. Unfortunately, the chemical instability at the N1 glycosidic bond in physiological conditions hampered the definition of cADPR molecular mechanism of action [12]. In this frame, efforts have been devoted to the synthesis of stable cADPR analogues [13–16]. In particular, the replacement of the adenine with hypoxanthine generated the very stable cIDPR analogue **2** which retained the same Ca^{2+} mobilizing activity of the endogenous metabolite [17]. In the last few years, we have produced both in solution [18–21] and on solid phase [22,23] some cIDPR analogues with alkyl chains in the place of the northern ribose (**3**–**7**). As we have found a promising Ca^{2+} mobilizing activity in the derivative with a pentyl chain (**6**, $n = 4$) in a neuronal cellular model [18], we have recently prepared a new flexible cIDPR analogue (**8**), with a 2″,3″-dihydroxypentyl chain replacing the northern ribose [21].

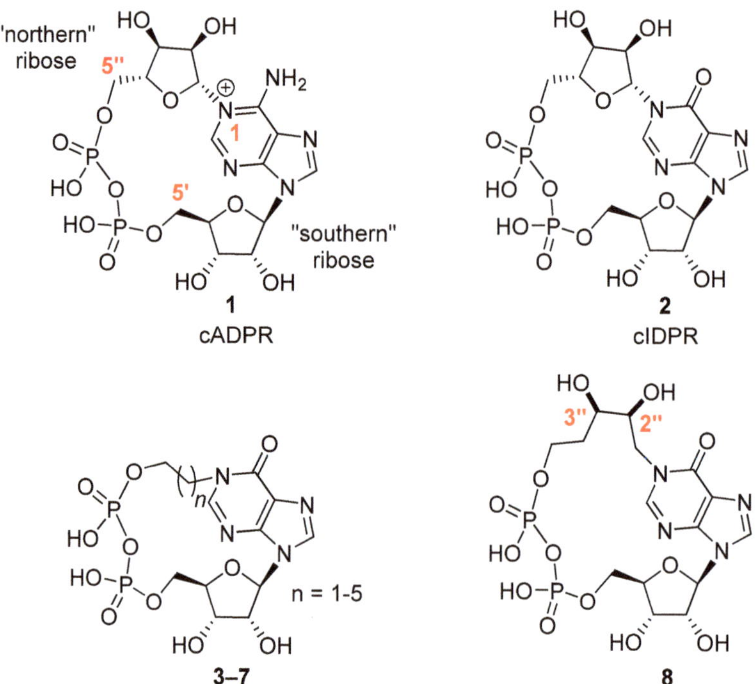

Figure 1. The structures of cADPR (**1**), cIDPR (**2**) and their analogues (**3**–**8**).

As the last mimic possesses the two OH groups in a ribose-like fashion, it may be considered the closest cIDPR flexible analogue. Interestingly, the cyclic compound **8** induced a concentration-dependent increase in $[Ca^{2+}]_i$ when perfused to primary cortical neurons as efficiently as cADPR.

Since 6-substituted purine nucleosides displayed interesting biological activities [24–26], herein we report on the synthesis and characterization of the O6-alkylated compound **9**, obtained as a side product during the coupling reaction of the protected inosine **10** and the tosylate **11** (Scheme 1). That reaction was revealed to be fundamental for the construction of the new cyclic analogue (**8**) scaffold.

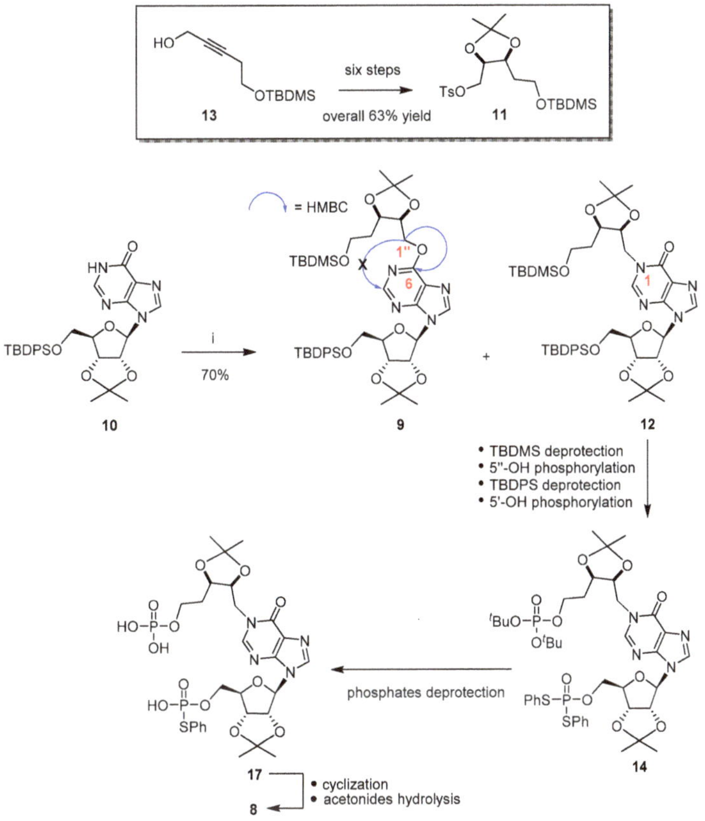

Scheme 1. Reagents and conditions: (i) **11**, DBU, DMF, 80 °C, 12 h (entry 6, Table 1).

Table 1. Optimization of the reaction between **10** and **11** [1].

Entry	Base	Equivalents [2]	Temperature (°C)	Yield (%)	9:12
1	K_2CO_3	1 or 3	r.t.	No reaction	-
2	K_2CO_3	3	80	10	20:80
3	Triethylamine	1 or 3	r.t.	No reaction	-
4	Triethylamine	3	80	No reaction	-
5	DBU	1 or 3	r.t.	No reaction	-
6	DBU	3	80	70	30:70
7	DBU	3	120	30	60:40

[1] All the reactions were carried out in anhydrous *N*,*N*-dimethylformamide (DMF) as solvent. [2] Calculated from **10**.

2. Results and Discussion

Scheme 1 shows the convergent synthetic approach that we have used for the preparation of the cyclic compound **8**. The ribose-protected inosine **10**, after reaction with the tosylate **11**, afforded as the main product the N1-alkylated derivative **12**. The electrophile **11** was prepared as a racemic mixture starting from the commercially available propargyl alcohol **13** with an overall 63% yield [21].

To obtain the target compound **8**, we used the well-known Hata protocol, which required an I_2 mediated cyclopyrophosphorylation reaction among a phosphomonoester and a phosphorothioate [14]. As a TBDMS group could be selectively removed in the presence of a TBDPS group [27], we followed the synthetic sequence reported in Scheme 1, and compound **14** was readily obtained. The two phosphates in **14** were then deprotected to give the key intermediate **17**. The pyrophosphate bond formation was carried out by adding compound **17** through a syringe pump to a very diluted solution of I_2. The cyclic compound was isolated from a complex reaction mixture and finally deprotected from both the acetonides, affording the new cADPR analogue **8** with an overall 1% yield.

The reaction between the protected inosine **10** with the electrophile **11** has been studied in detail. In principle, as hypoxanthine is an ambident nucleophile [28] at the N1 and O6 purine positions [29,30], the two regioisomers **12** and **9** could be expected. In our studies focused on the inosine N1 functionalization, we discovered that the Mitsunobu reaction was not a good method to regioselectivity obtain the N1-alkylated isomer. In fact, the reaction of inosine with di-*tert*-butyl (5-hydroxypentyl)phosphonate in the presence of diethyl azodicarboxylate (DEAD) and triphenylphosphine (PPh_3) afforded mainly the O6-alkylated regioisomer. We attributed the observed regioselectivity to the hard–hard interaction between the alkoxy-phosphonium cation intermediate and the nucleobase O6 atom [19]. On the other hand, previous findings demonstrated that inosine could be efficiently alkylated at the N1 purine position at room temperature (r.t.) when a soft electrophile was used [31]. Unfortunately, all the attempts to transform both the tosylate **11** and its primary alcohol precursor into the iodide derivative proceeded with very unsatisfactory yields [21]. As literature data reported on the efficient nucleophilic mediated displacement of a tosylate flanked by an isopropylidene under mild conditions [32,33], we reacted the inosine derivative **10** with the electrophile **11** at r.t. in the presence of some bases (Table 1); unfortunately, no reaction took place. By increasing the temperature, we noted on TLC (petroleum ether/AcOEt, 6:4) the formation of two spots. 1D/2D NMR analyses of the purified compounds (see Supplementary Materials) allowed to assign the N1-alkylated inosine **12** to the spot with Rf = 0.10, whereas the O6-alkylated inosine **9** to that with Rf = 0.50. In detail, in the ^{1}H NMR spectrum of compound **12** the two 1″-H protons resonated as two doublets of doublets centered at 4.70 and 4.66 ppm and correlated with their carbon atom resonating around 47.7 ppm. The HMBC correlation between the purine 2-H and the C1″ carbon atom supported the structure **12** [21]. Conversely, in the ^{1}H NMR spectrum of compound **9** (Figure S1, Supplementary Materials) the 1″-H protons resonated in the range 4.68–4.54 ppm and correlated with their carbon atom resonating at 65.6 ppm (Figure S4). The HMBC correlation between the two 1″-H protons and the C6 purine carbon atom resonating at 160.3 ppm and the absence of HMBC correlation between the purine 2-H (8.43 ppm) and the C1″ carbon atom supported the structure **9** (Figure S5).

Careful tuning of the reaction conditions allowed to recover the N1-alkylated regioisomer **12** as the main product. In particular, 3.0 equiv. of 1,8-diazabicyclo[5.4.0]undec-7-ene (DBU) and 80 °C for 12 h were the best conditions to recover the N1 and O6 regioisomers with a good 70% yield in a 7:3 ratio. (Scheme 2 and Table 1) Higher temperatures were detrimental to the reaction yield and increased the ratio **9**:**12**. The last experimental evidence could be explained assuming that compound **9** is the thermodynamic regioisomer.

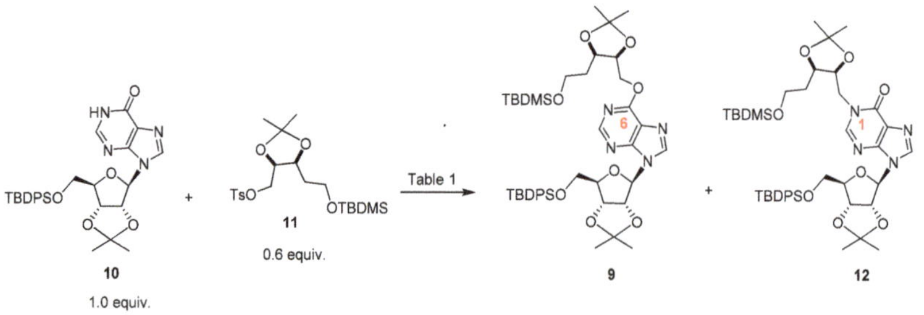

Scheme 2. The reaction of the nucleoside **10** with the tosylate **11**.

3. Materials and Methods

All the reagents and solvents were commercially available and used without further purification. ^{1}H- and ^{13}C-NMR spectra were acquired on the Bruker Avance 600 MHz spectrometer (Bruker-Biospin, Billerica, MA, USA) using $CDCl_3$ as solvent. NMR chemical shifts are reported in parts per million (δ) relative to residual solvents signals: $CHCl_3$ 7.26 for ^{1}H-NMR and $CDCl_3$ 77.0, for ^{13}C-NMR. The ^{1}H NMR chemical shifts were assigned through 2D NMR experiments. The NMR spectra were processed with the MestReNova (Mestrelab Research, Santiago de Campostela, Spain) suite. The HRESI-MS spectra were acquired on a Thermo Orbitrap XL mass spectrometer (Thermo Fisher Scientific, Waltham, MA, USA). Column chromatography was carried out on silica gel-60 (Merck, Readington Township, NJ, USA, 0.063–0.200 mm). TLC analyses were carried out on F_{254} silica gel plates (0.2 mm thick, Merck). TLC spots were detected under UV light (254 nm).

O6-[(2″,3″-*O*-isopropylidene-5″-*O*-*tert*-butyldimethylsilyl)pentyl]-5′-*O*-*tert*-butyldiphenylsilyl-2′,3′-*O*-isopropylideneinosine **9**. To a stirred solution of compound **10** (0.10 g, 0.18 mmol) in anhydrous DMF (2.0 mL), DBU (80 μL, 0.55 mmol) was added. After 20 min. the tosylate **11** (49 mg, 0.11 mmol) was added and reaction warmed to 80 °C for 12 h (TLC monitoring: petroleum ether/AcOEt, 6:4). The mixture was cooled, and the solvents removed under reduced pressure. The crude product was purified over a silica gel column eluted with increasing amounts of AcOEt in petroleum ether (up to 20%), giving the pure **9** as a 1:1 mixture of diastereomers (Rf = 0.50). Colorless syrup (21% yield). ^{1}H NMR (600 MHz, CD_3Cl) δ 8.43 (s, 1H, 2-H), 8.42 (s, 1H, 2-H), 8.07 (s, 1H, 8-H), 8.07 (s, 1H, 8-H), 7.62–7.54 (complex signal, 8H, arom.), 7.43–7.25 (complex signal, 12H, arom.), 6.15 (d, J = 1.7 Hz, 2H, 2 × 1′-H), 5.32–5.28 (m, 2H, 2 × 2′-H), 4.98–4.95 (m, 2H, 2 × 3′-H), 4.68–4.62 (m, 2H, 2 × 1″-H_a), 4.61–4.54 (complex signal, 4H, 2 × 1″-H_b and 2 × 2″-H), 4.49–4.43 (m, 2H, 2 × 3″-H), 4.42–4.38 (m, 2H, 2 × 4′-H), 3.92–3.85 (m, 2H, 2 × 5′-H_a), 3.83–3.74 (complex signal, 6H, 2 × 5′-H_b and 2 × 5″-$H_{a,b}$), 1.97–1.89 (m, 2H, 2 × 4″-H_a), 1.85–1.75 (m, 2H, 2 × 4″-H_b), 1.62 (s, 6H, 2 × CH_3 acetonide), 1.48 (s, 6H, 2 × CH_3 acetonide), 1.37 (two overlapped singlets, 12H, 4 × CH_3 acetonide), 1.01 (two overlapped singlets, 18H, 2 × ^{t}Bu), 0.88 (s, 18H, 2 × ^{t}Bu), 0.04 (s, 6H, 2 × $SiCH_3$), 0.05 (s, 6H, 2 × $SiCH_3$). ^{13}C NMR (151 MHz, $CDCl_3$) δ 160.32 (2 × C6), 152.10 (C2), 152.08 (C2), 151.45 (C4), 151.44 (C4), 141.01 (C8), 140.98 (C8), 135.49, 135.47, 132.82, 132.80, 132.69, 129.85, 127.74, 127.69, 127.62, 122.05 (2 × C5), 114.34 (C_q ribose acetonide) 114.33 (C_q ribose acetonide), 108.37 (2 × C_q acetonide), 91.19 (C1′), 91.17 (C1′), 87.02 (C4′), 86.97 (C4′), 84.40 (C2′), 84.36 (C2′), 81.36 (C3′), 81.35 (C3′), 75.14 (C2″), 75.12 (C2″), 73.71 (C3″), 73.70 (C3″), 65.60 (2 × C1″), 63.85 (2 × C5′), 60.02 (C5″), 60.00 (C5″), 32.16 (C4″), 32.14 (C4″), 29.66, 28.19, 28.17, 27.19, 26.81, 25.91, 25.86, 25.58, 25.35, 19.15, 18.30, −5.39, −5.44. HRESI-MS m/z 819.4184, ($[M + H]^+$ calcd. for $C_{43}H_{63}N_4O_8Si_2$ 819.4191).

4. Conclusions

Purine bases and nucleosides carrying O-, N- and C-substituents at the C6 position represent an important class of compounds endowed with important biological activities. These compounds are generally prepared by nucleophilic aromatic (S_NAr) substitutions, [34] metal-mediated cross-coupling reactions [35,36] and by Grignard's reagents addition [26] to 6-halopurine ribosides. In our search of new cADPR analogues, we have obtained the O6-alkylated inosine **9** as a side product during the S_N2 reaction between the nucleoside **10** and the tosylate **11**. The O6 reactivity of the ambident nucleophile hypoxanthine in **10** was a consequence of the high temperature necessary to perform the coupling reaction. Product **9** is an interesting intermediate that will be exploited for the synthesis of unprecedented O6-substituted cADPR derivatives.

Supplementary Materials: The following are available online. Figures S1–S6: copies of ^{1}H-, ^{13}C-NMR, COSY, HSQC, HMBC and HRESI-MS spectra of compound **9**.

Author Contributions: S.D. conceived and designed the experiments; V.P. performed the synthetic experiments; M.M. performed the spectroscopic experiments; M.T. and A.M. analyzed the data; R.N. finalized the draft; S.D. wrote the paper. All authors have read and agreed to the published version of the manuscript.

Funding: This work was funded by the institutional financial support to SYSBIO.ISBE.IT within the Italian Roadmap for ESFRI Research Infrastructures and by the PON-AIM RTDA_L1 (AIM 1873131-2).

Data Availability Statement: No data available.

Acknowledgments: The authors are grateful to Luisa Cuorvo for the technical assistance.

Conflicts of Interest: The authors declare no conflict of interest.

References

1. Borbone, N.; Piccialli, G.; Roviello, G.N.; Oliviero, G. Nucleoside analogues and nucleoside precursors as drugs in the fight against SARS-CoV-2 and other coronaviruses. *Molecules* **2021**, *26*, 986. [CrossRef] [PubMed]
2. Yates, M.K.; Seley-Radtke, K.L. The evolution of antiviral nucleoside analogues: A review for chemists and non-chemists. Part II: Complex modifications to the nucleoside scaffold. *Antivir. Res.* **2019**, *162*, 5–21. [CrossRef]
3. Guinan, M.; Benckendor, C.; Smith, M.; Miller, G.J.; Way, S.; Derek, J.; Mcphee, J. Evaluation Analogues Evaluation of Anticancer Anticancer Nucleoside. *Molecules* **2020**, *25*, 2050. [CrossRef]
4. Giuliani, A.L.; Sarti, A.C.; Di Virgilio, F. Extracellular nucleotides and nucleosides as signalling molecules. *Immunol. Lett.* **2019**, *205*, 16–24. [CrossRef] [PubMed]
5. Ewald, B.; Sampath, D.; Plunkett, W. Nucleoside analogues: Molecular mechanisms signaling cell death. *Oncogene* **2008**, *27*, 6522–6537. [CrossRef] [PubMed]
6. Zarrilli, F.; Amato, F.; Morgillo, C.M.C.M.; Pinto, B.; Santarpia, G.; Borbone, N.; D'Errico, S.; Catalanotti, B.; Piccialli, G.; Castaldo, G.; et al. Peptide nucleic acids as miRNA target protectors for the treatment of cystic fibrosis. *Molecules* **2017**, *22*, 1144. [CrossRef] [PubMed]
7. Poppe, H.; Rybalkin, S.D.; Rehmann, H.; Hinds, T.R.; Tang, X.B.; Christensen, A.E.; Schwede, F.; Genieser, H.G.; Bos, J.L.; Doskeland, S.O.; et al. Cyclic nucleotide analogues as probes of signaling pathways. *Nat. Methods* **2008**, *5*, 277–278. [CrossRef] [PubMed]
8. Fajardo, A.M.; Piazza, G.A.; Tinsley, H.N. The role of cyclic nucleotide signaling pathways in cancer: Targets for prevention and treatment. *Cancers* **2014**, *6*, 436–458. [CrossRef] [PubMed]
9. Clapper, D.L.; Walseth, T.F.; Dargie, P.J.; Lee, H.C. Pyridine nucleotide metabolites stimulate calcium release from sea urchin egg microsomes desensitized to inositol trisphosphate. *J. Biol. Chem.* **1987**, *262*, 9561–9568. [CrossRef]
10. Guse, A.H. Calcium mobilizing second messengers derived from NAD. *Biochim. Biophys. Acta* **2015**, *1854*, 1132–1137. [CrossRef]
11. Gul, R.; Park, J.H.; Kim, S.Y.; Jang, K.Y.; Chae, J.K.; Ko, J.K.; Kim, U.H. Inhibition of ADP-ribosyl cyclase attenuates angiotensin II-induced cardiac hypertrophy. *Cardiovasc. Res.* **2009**, *81*, 582–591. [CrossRef] [PubMed]
12. Potter, B.V.L.; Walseth, T.F. Medicinal chemistry and pharmacology of cyclic ADP-ribose. *Curr. Mol. Med.* **2004**, *4*, 303–311. [CrossRef] [PubMed]
13. Takano, S.; Tsuzuki, T.; Murayama, T.; Kameda, T.; Kumaki, Y.; Sakurai, T.; Fukuda, H.; Watanabe, M.; Arisawa, M.; Shuto, S. Synthesis of 8-Substituted Analogues of Cyclic ADP-4-Thioribose and Their Unexpected Identification as Ca^{2+}-Mobilizing Full Agonists. *J. Med. Chem.* **2017**, *60*, 5868–5875. [CrossRef]
14. Watt, J.M.; Graeff, R.; Thomas, M.P.; Potter, B.V.L. Second messenger analogues highlight unexpected substrate sensitivity of CD38: Total synthesis of the hybrid "l-cyclic inosine 5′-diphosphate ribose". *Sci. Rep.* **2017**, *7*, 16100. [CrossRef]
15. Sato, T.; Watanabe, M.; Tsuzuki, T.; Takano, S.; Murayama, T.; Sakurai, T.; Kameda, T.; Fukuda, H.; Arisawa, M.; Shuto, S. Design, Synthesis, and Identification of 4″α-Azidoethyl-cyclic ADP-Carbocyclic-ribose as a Highly Potent Analogue of Cyclic ADP-Ribose, a Ca^{2+}-Mobilizing Second Messenger. *J. Med. Chem.* **2016**, *59*, 7282–7286. [CrossRef] [PubMed]
16. Galeone, A.; Mayol, L.; Oliviero, G.; Piccialli, G.; Varra, M. Synthesis of a novel N-1 carbocyclic, N-9 butyl analogue of cyclic ADP ribose (cADPR). *Tetrahedron* **2002**, *58*, 363–368. [CrossRef]
17. Wagner, G.K.; Guse, A.H.; Potter, B.V.L. Rapid synthetic route toward structurally modified derivatives of cyclic adenosine 5′-diphosphate ribose. *J. Org. Chem.* **2005**, *70*, 4810–4819. [CrossRef] [PubMed]
18. Mahal, A.; D'Errico, S.; Borbone, N.; Pinto, B.; Secondo, A.; Costantino, V.; Tedeschi, V.; Oliviero, G.; Piccialli, V.; Piccialli, G. Synthesis of cyclic N^1-pentylinosine phosphate, a new structurally reduced cADPR analogue with calcium-mobilizing activity on PC12 cells. *Beilstein J. Org. Chem.* **2015**, *11*, 2689–2695. [CrossRef]
19. D'Errico, S.; Borbone, N.; Catalanotti, B.; Secondo, A.; Petrozziello, T.; Piccialli, I.; Pannaccione, A.; Costantino, V.; Mayol, L.; Piccialli, G.; et al. Synthesis and Biological Evaluation of a New Structural Simplified Analogue of cADPR, a Calcium-Mobilizing Secondary Messenger Firstly Isolated from Sea Urchin Eggs. *Mar. Drugs* **2018**, *16*, 89. [CrossRef]
20. D'Errico, S.; Basso, E.; Falanga, A.P.A.P.; Marzano, M.; Pozzan, T.; Piccialli, V.; Piccialli, G.; Oliviero, G.; Borbone, N. New linear precursors of cIDPR derivatives as stable analogues of cADPR: A potent second messenger with Ca^{2+}-Modulating activity isolated from sea urchin eggs. *Mar. Drugs* **2019**, *17*, 476. [CrossRef]
21. D'Errico, S.; Greco, F.; Patrizia Falanga, A.; Tedeschi, V.; Piccialli, I.; Marzano, M.; Terracciano, M.; Secondo, A.; Roviello, G.N.; Oliviero, G.; et al. Probing the Ca^{2+} mobilizing properties on primary cortical neurons of a new stable cADPR mimic. *Bioorg. Chem.* **2021**, *117*, 105401. [CrossRef]

22. Oliviero, G.; D'Errico, S.; Borbone, N.; Amato, J.; Piccialli, V.; Varra, M.; Piccialli, G.; Mayol, L. A solid-phase approach to the synthesis of N-1-alkyl analogues of cyclic inosine-diphosphate-ribose (cIDPR). *Tetrahedron* **2010**, *66*, 1931–1936. [CrossRef]
23. D'Errico, S.; Oliviero, G.; Borbone, N.; Amato, J.; Piccialli, V.; Varra, M.; Mayol, L.; Piccialli, G. Solid-phase synthesis of a new diphosphate 5-aminoimidazole-4-carboxamide riboside (AICAR) derivative and studies toward cyclic AICAR diphosphate ribose. *Molecules* **2011**, *16*, 8110–8118. [CrossRef]
24. Bonnac, L.F.; Dreis, C.D.; Geraghty, R.J. Structure activity relationship, 6-modified purine riboside analogues to activate hSTING, stimulator of interferon genes. *Bioorgan. Med. Chem. Lett.* **2019**, 126819. [CrossRef] [PubMed]
25. Hulpia, F.; Bouton, J.; Campagnaro, G.D.; Alfayez, I.A.; Mabille, D.; Maes, L.; de Koning, H.P.; Caljon, G.; Van Calenbergh, S. C6–O-alkylated 7-deazainosine nucleoside analogues: Discovery of potent and selective anti-sleeping sickness agents. *Eur. J. Med. Chem.* **2020**, *188*, 112018. [CrossRef] [PubMed]
26. D'Errico, S.; Oliviero, G.; Amato, J.; Borbone, N.; Cerullo, V.; Hemminki, A.; Piccialli, V.; Zaccaria, S.; Mayol, L.; Piccialli, G. Synthesis and biological evaluation of unprecedented ring-expanded nucleosides (RENs) containing the imidazo[4,5-d][1,2,6]oxadiazepine ring system. *Chem. Commun.* **2012**, *48*, 9310–9312. [CrossRef] [PubMed]
27. Prakash, C.; Saleh, S.; Blair, I.A. Selective Deprotection of Silyl Ethers. *Tetrahedron Lett.* **1989**, *30*, 19–22. [CrossRef]
28. Leškovskis, K.; Zaķis, J.M.; Novosjolova, I.; Turks, M. Applications of Purine Ring Opening in the Synthesis of Imidazole, Pyrimidine, and New Purine Derivatives. *Eur. J. Org. Chem.* **2021**, *2021*, 5027–5052. [CrossRef]
29. Shuto, S.; Shirato, M.; Sumita, Y.; Ueno, Y.; Matsuda, A. Nucleosides and Nucleotides. 173. Synthesis of Cyclic IDP-carbocyclic-ribose, a Stable Mimic of Cyclic ADP-Ribose. Significant Facilitation of the Intramolecular Condensation Reaction of N-1-(Carbocyclic-ribosyl)inosine 5″, 6″-Diphosphate Derivatives by an 8-Bromo-Sustitution at the Hypoxanthine Moiety. *J. Org. Chem.* **1998**, *63*, 1986–1994.
30. De Napoli, L.; Di Fabio, G.; Messere, A.; Montesarchio, D.; Piccialli, G.; Varra, M. Synthetic studies on the glycosylation of the base residues of inosine and uridine. *J. Chem. Soc. Perkin Trans.* **1999**, *1*, 3489–3493. [CrossRef]
31. Hyde, R.M.; Broom, A.D.; Buckheit, R.W. Antiviral amphipathic oligo- and polyribonucleotides: Analogue development and biological studies. *J. Med. Chem.* **2003**, *46*, 1878–1885. [CrossRef] [PubMed]
32. Karnekanti, R.; Hanumaiah, M.; Sharma, G.V.M. Stereoselective Total Synthesis of (+)-Anamarine and 8-epi-(-)-Anamarine from D-Mannitol. *Synthesis* **2015**, *47*, 2997–3008. [CrossRef]
33. Lanier, M.L.; Park, H.; Mukherjee, P.; Timmerman, J.C.; Ribeiro, A.A.; Widenhoefer, R.A.; Hong, J. Formal Synthesis of (+)-Laurencin by Gold(I)-Catalyzed Intramolecular Dehydrative Alkoxylation. *Chem.-A Eur. J.* **2017**, *23*, 7180–7184. [CrossRef] [PubMed]
34. Véliz, E.A.; Beal, P.A. 6-Bromopurine nucleosides as reagents for nucleoside analogue synthesis. *J. Org. Chem.* **2001**, *66*, 8592–8598. [CrossRef] [PubMed]
35. Buchanan, H.S.; Pauff, S.M.; Kosmidis, T.D.; Taladriz-Sender, A.; Rutherford, O.I.; Hatit, M.Z.C.; Fenner, S.; Watson, A.J.B.; Burley, G.A. Modular, Step-Efficient Palladium-Catalyzed Cross-Coupling Strategy to Access C6-Heteroaryl 2-Aminopurine Ribonucleosides. *Org. Lett.* **2017**, *19*, 3759–3762. [CrossRef] [PubMed]
36. Perkins, J.J.; Shurtleff, V.W.; Johnson, A.M.; El Marrouni, A. Synthesis of C6-Substituted Purine Nucleoside Analogues via Late-Stage Photoredox/Nickel Dual Catalytic Cross-Coupling. *ACS Med. Chem. Lett.* **2021**, *12*, 662–666. [CrossRef] [PubMed]

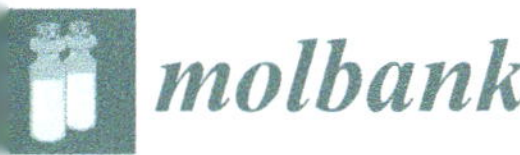 molbank

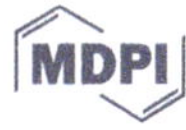

Short Note

Dichloro{4-(4-chlorophenoxy)phthalazin-1-yl}methylphosphonic dichloride

Dyhia Amrane [1], Omar Khoumeri [1], Patrice Vanelle [1,2,*] and Nicolas Primas [1,2,*]

[1] Aix Marseille Univ, CNRS, ICR UMR 7273, Equipe Pharmaco-Chimie Radicalaire, Faculté de Pharmacie, CEDEX 05, 13385 Marseille, France

[2] APHM, Hôpital Conception, Service Central de la Qualité et de l'Information Pharmaceutiques, 13005 Marseille, France

* Correspondence: patrice.vanelle@univ-amu.fr (P.V.); nicolas.primas@univ-amu.fr (N.P.)

Abstract: As part of our ongoing scaffold-hopping work on an antiplasmodial 2-trichloromethylquinazoline scaffold, we aimed to explore the 1-trichloromethylphthalazine scaffold as a potential new antimalarial series. Using previously chlorination conditions described by our lab to obtain a trichloromethyl group from a methyl group, we did not obtain the target compound; instead, we obtained a dichloro methylphosphonic dichloride side product **3**. The nature of this compound was then characterized by NMR, HRMS and X-ray crystallography. The same issue was previously reported by Kato et al., starting from the 2-methyl-3-nitropyridine. Finally, compound **3,** although not cytotoxic, was not active against *P. falciparum*, the parasite responsible for human malaria.

Keywords: phthalazine; chlorination; side product; phosphonic dichloride; *P. falciparum*; HepG2

Citation: Amrane, D.; Khoumeri, O.; Vanelle, P.; Primas, N. Dichloro{4-(4-chlorophenoxy)phthalazin-1-yl}methylphosphonic dichloride. *Molbank* **2022**, *2022*, M1439. https://doi.org/10.3390/M1439

Academic Editors: Stefano D'Errico and Annalisa Guaragna

Received: 12 August 2022
Accepted: 2 September 2022
Published: 5 September 2022

Publisher's Note: MDPI stays neutral with regard to jurisdictional claims in published maps and institutional affiliations.

1. Introduction

Malaria is still the leading cause of mortality in comparison to other parasitic diseases. In 2020, malaria deaths dramatically increased by 12% from 2019 to an estimated 627,000, among which 77% were children under 5 years old: this was mainly due to service disruptions during the COVID-19 pandemic. [1] To overcome the resistance of the causal agent *Plasmodium* to most of the marketed therapies, including the most recent ones such as artemisinin-combination therapies (ACTs), a huge effort has been made to highlight new derivatives active against *Plasmodium* and display original mechanisms of action [2]. With the aim of developing new antiplasmodial compounds, our laboratory explored different aza-heterocyclic scaffolds bearing a trichloromethyl group, which was mandatory for providing the antiparasitic activity [3–5]. We previously obtained a hit molecule in the 2-trichloromethylquinazoline series bearing a 4′-chlorophenoxy substituent at position 4, showing micromolar activity against *P. falciparum* and a low cytotoxicity against the human HepG2 cell line [6] (Figure 1).

W2 *P. falciparum* EC_{50} = 1.1 µM
HepG2 CC_{50} = 50 µM
SI = 45

Figure 1. Previously described antiplasmodial Hit A.

In order to continue the pharmacomodulation work around this aza-heterocyclic scaffold, we performed a scaffold-hopping strategy using ring variation, among which we explored the phthalazine moiety. Indeed, phthalazines have recently gained some importance as privileged scaffolds in bioactive compounds, such as anticancer drugs, namely Olaparib [7] and Vatalanib [8], as well as the antihistaminic H_1 drug Azelastine [9] (Figure 2). Numerous other bioactive molecules are currently in development in various therapeutic areas [10].

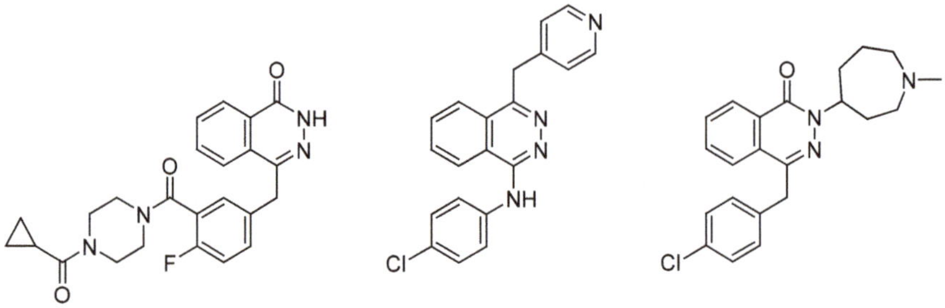

Olaparib Vatalanib Azelastine

Figure 2. Some drugs based on phthalazine moiety.

2. Results

To obtain the target compound **B**, we followed our previously described reaction condition applied to the phthalazine scaffold (Scheme 1). Starting from the readily accessible 1-chloro-4-methylphthalazine **1** [11], we first introduced an S_NAr reaction to the 4-chlorophenoxy substituent at position 1, using the appropriate phenol and cesium carbonate as a base to yield **2** (71%). Then, we performed the chlorination reaction in order to obtain the 4-trichloromethyl group from the 4-methyl group, using a mixture of PCl_5 in $POCl_3$. This reaction is usually performed under microwave heating, which allows for the best yields in a short reaction time [12].

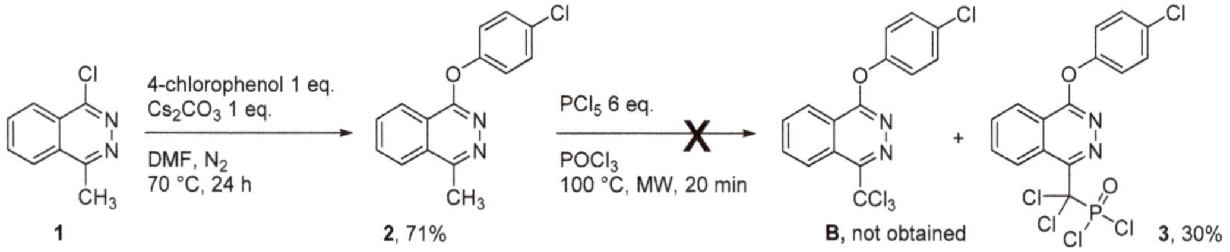

4-chlorophenol 1 eq.
Cs_2CO_3 1 eq.
DMF, N_2
70 °C, 24 h
PCl_5 6 eq.
$POCl_3$
100 °C, MW, 20 min
1 **2**, 71% **B**, not obtained **3**, 30%

Scheme 1. Reaction conditions for the synthesis of compound **B** and structure of compound **3**.

A mixture of two compounds was obtained. Usually, the reaction leads to a mixture of the target compound -CCl_3 and the dichlorinated intermediate -$CHCl_2$. However, in our study, we noticed the formation of a new unexpected compound following the purification step. After complementary unambiguous analyses, we confirmed by NMR, HRMS and X-ray crystallography (Figure 3) [13] that this compound was dichloro{4-(4-chlorophenoxy)phthalazin-1-yl}methylphosphonic dichloride **3** (Scheme 1) (see Supplementary data).

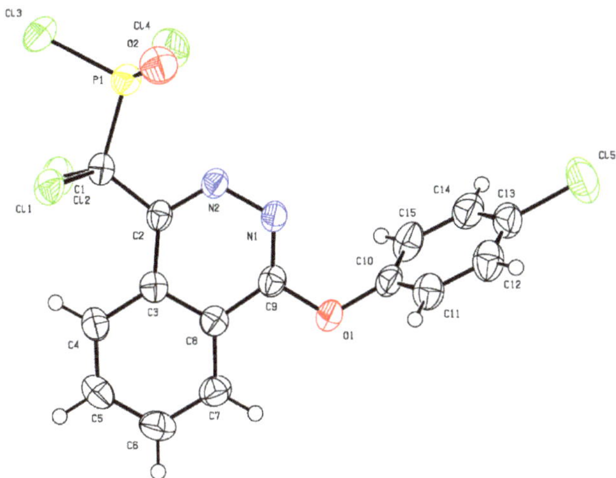

Figure 3. X-ray crystallography structure of compound **3**.

3. Discussion

After conducting bibliographical research, we noticed that Kato et al. previously reported the formation of a similar unwanted compound upon the chlorination of 2-methyl-3-nitropyridine using a mixture of PCl_5 in $POCl_3$, leading to dichloro-(3-nitro-2-pyridyl)methylphosphonic dichloride [14] (Scheme 2).

Finally, we wanted to explore the biological potential of **3**: this compound was not active against *P. falciparum* (EC_{50} = 28.9 μM), nor was it cytotoxic on the HepG2 cell line (CC_{50} = 62.5 μM).

NO_2 / CH_3 / N — PCl_5 6 eq. / $POCl_3$ / 100 °C, MW, 20 min → NO_2 / O / P–Cl / Cl / N / Cl Cl / 34%

Scheme 2. Similar issue observed by Kato et al. [14] in pyridine series.

Several factors could explain the direct phosphonylation of methylphthalazine **2**, although the mechanism of the reaction is not clearly established:

(1) The substituent effect of the 4-chlorophenoxy group to the nucleophilic behavior of the 1-methyl group;

(2) The ability of the phthalazine to form a complex with the strongest available electrophile, i.e., PCl_5, if sterically possible.

The chlorination by PCl_5 is usually favored, thanks to a lower enthalpy of activation; however, it is sterically more constrained than phosphonylation by $POCl_3$, because oxygen atoms are much smaller than chlorine atoms [14]. Thus, PCl_5 cannot react due to its size, but $POCl_3$ can come close enough to react with the nucleophilic carbon, giving the intermediate phosphonic dichloride. The next step could involve intramolecular chlorination to give the monochlorophosphonic dichloride. Repeating the chlorination step finally gave the product **3** (Scheme 3).

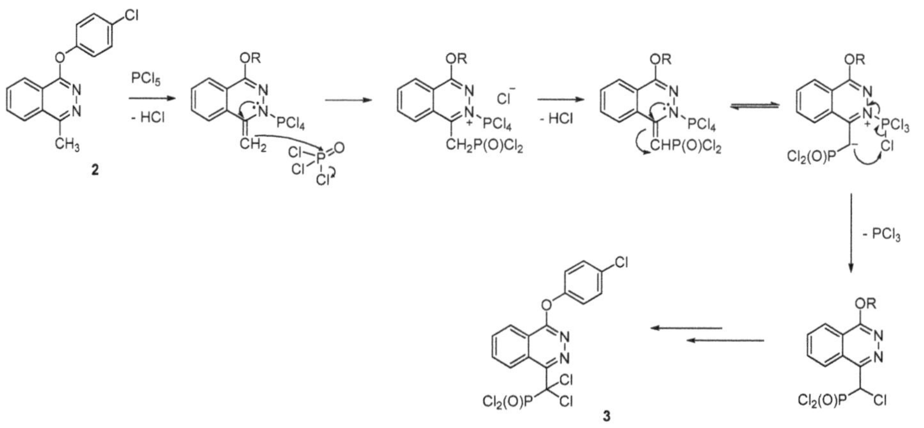

Scheme 3. Hypothesized reaction mechanism.

4. Materials and Methods

Melting points were determined on a Köfler melting point apparatus (Wagner & Munz GmbH, München, Germany) and were uncorrected. Elemental analyses were carried out at the Spectropole, Faculté des Sciences de Saint-Jêrome (Marseille) with a Thermo Finnigan EA1112 analyzer (Thermo Finnigan, San Jose, CA, USA). NMR spectra were recorded on a Bruker Avance NEO 400MHz NanoBay spectrometer at the Faculté de Pharmacie of Marseille (^{1}H NMR: reference $CDCl_3$ δ = 7.26 ppm and ^{13}C NMR: reference $CHCl_3$ δ = 76.9 ppm). The following adsorbent was used for column chromatography: silica gel 60 (Merck KGaA, Darmstadt, Germany, particle size 0.063–0.200 mm, 70–230 mesh ASTM). TLC was performed on 5 cm × 10 cm aluminum plates coated with silica gel 60F-254 (Merck) in an appropriate eluent. Visualization was performed with ultraviolet light (234 nm). The purity of synthesized compounds was checked by LC/MS analyses, which were performed at the Faculté de Pharmacie of Marseille with a Thermo Scientific Accela High Speed LC System® (Waltham, MA, USA), coupled to a single quadrupole mass spectrometer Thermo MSQ Plus®. The RP-HPLC column was a Thermo Hypersil Gold® 50 × 2.1 mm (C18 bounded), with particles of a diameter of 1.9 mm. The volume of sample injected on the column was 1 µL. The chromatographic analysis with a total duration of 8 min, was performed on the following solvents' gradients: t = 0 min, methanol/water 50:50; 0 < t < 4 min, linear increase in the proportion of methanol to a methanol/water ratio of 95:5; 4 < t < 6 min, methanol/water 95:5; 6 < t < 7 min, linear decrease in the proportion of methanol to return to a methanol/water ratio of 50:50; 6 < t< 7 min, methanol/water 50:50. The water used was buffered with ammonium acetate 5 mM. The flow rate of the mobile phase was 0.3 mL/min. The retention times (t_R) of the molecules analyzed were indicated in min. The microwave reactions were performed using multimode reactor ETHOS Synth Lab station (Ethos start, MLS GmbH, Leutkirch, Germany) in an open vessel with a power output of 0 to 800 W. Reagents were purchased and used without further purifications from Sigma-Aldrich or Fluorochem.

1-(4-Chlorophenoxy)-4-methylphthalazine (**2**). To a solution of 1-chloro-4-methylphthalazine (**1**) [11], (500 mg, 2.8 mmol) and 4-chlorophenol (360 mg, 2.8 mmol, 1.0 equiv) in anhydrous DMF (5 mL), Cs_2CO_3 (912 mg, 2.8 mmol, 1.0 equiv) was added under an inert atmosphere. The mixture was stirred at 70 °C for 24 h. After completion of the reaction, water was added, leading to a precipitate which was separated by filtration. The resulting yellow precipitate was then thoroughly washed with water. The precipitate was dissolved in CH_2Cl_2 and dried with Na_2SO_4. After filtration and evaporation, the resulting solid was purified by silica-gel column chromatography (Petroleum ether/CH_2Cl_2, 1:1 *v/v*) to afford the desired compound **2**.

Yield 71% (540 mg). Yellow solid. Mp 132–133 °C. ^{1}H NMR (400 MHz, $CDCl_3$) δ 8.46–8.34 (m, 1H), 8.08–8.02 (m, 1H), 8.00–7.93 (m, 2H), 7.39 (d, J = 8.9 Hz, 2H), 7.27 (d, J = 8.9 Hz, 2H), 2.93 (s, 3H). ^{13}C NMR (101 MHz, $CDCl_3$) δ 160.7, 155.1, 152.1, 132.9, 132.5, 130.6, 129.7, 129.1, 124.9, 123.6, 123.2, 119.9, 19.5. LC-MS (ESI+) t_R 5.42 min; m/z $[M+H]^+$ 271.11/273.12. HRMS (ESI): m/z calcd. for $C_{15}H_{12}ClN_2O$ $[M + H]^+$ 271.0633. Found: 271.0632.

Dichloro(4-(4-chlorophenoxy)phthalazin-1-yl)methyl)phosphonic dichloride (**3**). To a solution of 1-(4-Chlorophenoxy)-4-methylphthalazine (**2**) (500 mg, 1.85 mmol) in $POCl_3$ (10 mL) PCl_5 was added (2.31 g, 11.1 mmol). The reaction mixture was heated by a microwave reactor at a reflux of POCl3 for 20 min at 800 W. After cooling down, the reaction mixture was poured into ice, and then the pH was adjusted to neutrality with Na_2CO_3. The resulting solution was extracted three times with CH_2Cl_2. The organic phase was then washed with brine, dried over anhydrous $MgSO_4$, filtered and concentrated in a vacuum to afford the crude product, which was purified by silica-gel flash chromatography (using dichloromethane/petroleum ether from 5/5 to 7/3 v/v) to afford compound **3**.

Yield 30% (250 mg). Yellow solid. Mp 250 °C (degradation). ^{1}H NMR (400 MHz, $CDCl_3$) δ 8.75 (d, J = 7.9 Hz, 1H), 8.55 (d, J = 7.9 Hz, 1H), 8.10–8.06 (m, 2H), 7.42 (d, J = 8.5 Hz, 2H), 7.27 (d, J = 8.5 Hz, 2H). ^{13}C NMR (101 MHz, $CDCl_3$) δ 162.3, 151.6, 151.2, 133.4, 133.3, 131.6, 130.0, 126.1, 126.0, 125.2, 124.6, 123.3, 121.5. ^{31}P NMR (162 MHz, $CDCl_3$) δ 35.73. HRMS (ESI): m/z calcd. for $C_{15}H_9Cl_5N_2O_2P$ $[M + H]^+$ 456.8810. Found: 456.8806.

Crystal Data for $C_{15}H_8Cl_5N_2O_2P$ (M = 456.45 g/mol): monoclinic, space group $P2_1/n$ (no. 14), a = 7.9208(3) Å, b = 23.1270(9) Å, c = 9.9621(5) Å, β = 96.368(4)°, V = 1813.64(13) $Å^3$, Z = 4, T = 295 K, μ(MoKα) = 0.900 mm^{-1}, $Dcalc$ = 1.672 g/cm^3, 15,418 reflections measured (6.244° $\leq 2\Theta \leq$ 56.808°), 3992 unique (R_{int} = 0.0343, R_{sigma} = 0.0295), which were used in all calculations. The final R_1 was 0.0400 (I > 2σ(I)) and wR_2 was 0.1021 (all data).

Supplementary Materials: The following are available online: Figure S1, ^{1}H NMR spectra of 1-(4-Chlorophenoxy)-4-methylphthalazine; Figure S2, ^{13}C NMR spectra of 1-(4-Chlorophenoxy)-4-methylphthalazine; Figure S3, HRMS (ESI) spectra of 1-(4-Chlorophenoxy)-4-methylphthalazine; Figure S4, ^{1}H NMR spectra of Dichloro(4-(4-chlorophenoxy)phthalazin-1-yl)methyl)phosphonic dichloride; Figure S5, ^{13}C NMR spectra of Dichloro(4-(4-chlorophenoxy)phthalazin-1-yl)methyl)phosphonic dichloride; Figure S6, ^{31}P NMR spectra of Dichloro(4-(4-chlorophenoxy)phthalazin-1-yl)methyl)phosphonic dichloride; Figure S7, HRMS (ESI) spectra of Dichloro(4-(4-chlorophenoxy)phthalazin-1-yl)methyl)phosphonic dichloride.

Author Contributions: Funding acquisition, N.P.; investigation, D.A. and O.K.; methodology, D.A. and O.K.; supervision, P.V. and N.P.; writing—original draft, D.A. and N.P.; writing—review and editing, D.A., P.V. and N.P. All authors have read and agreed to the published version of the manuscript.

Funding: This research work was supported by a public grant of the French National Research Agency (Agence Nationale de la Recherche ANR), project NINTARMAL, grant number: ANR-17-CE11-0017.

Institutional Review Board Statement: Not applicable.

Informed Consent Statement: Not applicable.

Data Availability Statement: The X-ray data are deposited at CCDC as stated above.

Acknowledgments: The authors thank Michel Giorgi for his help in the determination of the crystal structure. The authors thank Aix-Marseille Université and the CNRS for their financial support.

Conflicts of Interest: The authors declare no conflict of interest. The funders had no role in the design of the study; in the collection, analyses, or interpretation of data; in the writing of the manuscript, or in the decision to publish the results.

Sample Availability: Samples of the compounds are available from the authors.

References

1. *World Malaria Report 2021*; World Health Organization: Geneva, Switzerland, 2021.
2. Burrows, J.N.; Duparc, S.; Gutteridge, W.E.; Hooft van Huijsduijnen, R.; Kaszubska, W.; Macintyre, F.; Mazzuri, S.; Möhrle, J.J.; Wells, T.N.C. New developments in anti-malarial target candidate and product profiles. *Malar. J.* **2017**, *16*, 26. [CrossRef] [PubMed]
3. Amrane, D.; Gellis, A.; Hutter, S.; Prieri, M.; Verhaeghe, P.; Azas, N.; Vanelle, P.; Primas, N. Synthesis and Antiplasmodial Evaluation of 4-Carboxamido- and 4-Alkoxy-2-Trichloromethyl Quinazolines. *Molecules* **2020**, *25*, 3929. [CrossRef] [PubMed]
4. Amrane, D.; Arnold, C.-S.; Hutter, S.; Sanz-Serrano, J.; Collia, M.; Azqueta, A.; Paloque, L.; Cohen, A.; Amanzougaghene, N.; Tajeri, S.; et al. 2-Phenoxy-3-Trichloromethylquinoxalines Are Antiplasmodial Derivatives with Activity against the Apicoplast of Plasmodium Falciparum. *Pharmaceuticals* **2021**, *14*, 724. [CrossRef] [PubMed]
5. Amrane, D.; Primas, N.; Arnold, C.-S.; Hutter, S.; Louis, B.; Sanz-Serrano, J.; Azqueta, A.; Amanzougaghene, N.; Tajeri, S.; Mazier, D.; et al. Antiplasmodial 2-Thiophenoxy-3-Trichloromethyl Quinoxalines Target the Apicoplast of Plasmodium Falciparum. *Eur. J. Med. Chem.* **2021**, *224*, 113722. [CrossRef] [PubMed]
6. Castera-Ducros, C.; Azas, N.; Verhaeghe, P.; Hutter, S.; Garrigue, P.; Dumètre, A.; Mbatchi, L.; Laget, M.; Remusat, V.; Sifredi, F.; et al. Targeting the Human Malaria Parasite Plasmodium Falciparum: In Vitro Identification of a New Antiplasmodial Hit in 4-Phenoxy-2-Trichloromethylquinazoline Series. *Eur. J. Med. Chem.* **2011**, *46*, 4184–4191. [CrossRef] [PubMed]
7. Robson, M.; Im, S.-A.; Senkus, E.; Xu, B.; Domchek, S.M.; Masuda, N.; Delaloge, S.; Li, W.; Tung, N.; Armstrong, A.; et al. Olaparib for Metastatic Breast Cancer in Patients with a Germline BRCA Mutation. *N. Engl. J. Med.* **2017**, *377*, 523–533. [CrossRef] [PubMed]
8. Scott, E.; Meinhardt, G.; Jacques, C.; Laurent, D.; Thomas, A.L. Vatalanib: The Clinical Development of a Tyrosine Kinase Inhibitor of Angiogenesis in Solid Tumours. *Expert Opin. Investig. Drugs* **2007**, *16*, 367–379. [CrossRef] [PubMed]
9. Ratner, P.H.; Findlay, S.R.; Hampel, F.; van Bavel, J.; Widlitz, M.D.; Freitag, J.J. A Double-Blind, Controlled Trial to Assess the Safety and Efficacy of Azelastine Nasal Spray in Seasonal Allergic Rhinitis. *J. Allergy Clin. Immunol.* **1994**, *94*, 818–825. [CrossRef]
10. Zaib, S.; Khan, I. Synthetic and Medicinal Chemistry of Phthalazines: Recent Developments, Opportunities and Challenges. *Bioorg. Chem.* **2020**, *105*, 104425. [CrossRef]
11. Elmeligie, S.; Aboul-Magd, A.M.; Lasheen, D.S.; Ibrahim, T.M.; Abdelghany, T.M.; Khojah, S.M.; Abouzid, K.A.M. Design and Synthesis of Phthalazine-Based Compounds as Potent Anticancer Agents with Potential Antiangiogenic Activity via VEGFR-2 Inhibition. *J. Enzyme Inhib. Med. Chem.* **2019**, *34*, 1347–1367. [CrossRef] [PubMed]
12. Verhaeghe, P.; Rathelot, P.; Gellis, A.; Rault, S.; Vanelle, P. Highly Efficient Microwave Assisted α-Trichlorination Reaction of α-Methylated Nitrogen Containing Heterocycles. *Tetrahedron* **2006**, *62*, 8173–8176. [CrossRef]
13. Primas, N.; Vanelle, P.; Amrane, D. CCDC 2074292: Experimental Crystal Structure Determination. 2021. Available online: https://www.ccdc.cam.ac.uk/structures/search?id=doi:10.5517/ccdc.csd.cc27mgn0&sid=DataCite (accessed on 11 August 2022).
14. Kato, T.; Katagiri, N.; Wagai, A. Synthesis of Methylpyridine Derivatives—XXXIII Phosphonylation and Chlorination of Methylpyridine and 3-Nitro-Methylpyridine Derivatives. *Tetrahedron* **1978**, *34*, 3445–3449. [CrossRef]

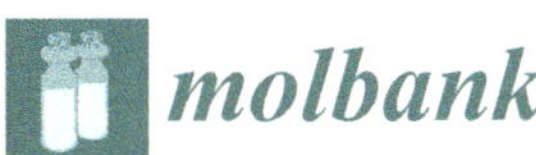 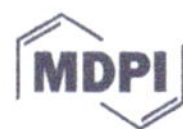

Short Note

19β,28-Epoxy-18α-olean-3β-ol-2-furoate from Allobetulin (19β,28-Epoxy-18α-olean-3β-ol)

Fulgentius Nelson Lugemwa

Department of Chemistry, Pennsylvania State University-York, 1031 Edgecomb Avenue, York, PA 17403, USA; ful4@psu.edu; Tel.: +1-717-771-8409

Abstract: The E ring of betulin rearranges and forms a cyclic ether when treated with an acid. Treatment of betulin with iodine generated hydrogen iodide in situ, which went on to promote the rearrangement at C-19 and C-20, followed by cyclization to form allobetulin. A reaction of allobetulin with 2-furoyl chloride yielded 19β,28-Epoxy-18α-olean-3β-ol-2-furoate.

Keywords: 19β,28-Epoxy-18α-olean-3β-ol-2-furoate; betulin; allobetulin; iodine; 2-furoyl chloride; esterification

Citation: Lugemwa, F.N. 19β,28-Epoxy-18α-olean-3β-ol-2-furoate from Allobetulin (19β,28-Epoxy-18α-olean-3β-ol). *Molbank* **2022**, *2022*, M1499. https://doi.org/10.3390/M1499

Academic Editors: Stefano D'Errico and Annalisa Guaragna

Received: 14 October 2022
Accepted: 10 November 2022
Published: 18 November 2022

1. Introduction

Betulin (lup-20(29)-ene-3β,28-diol), a pentacyclic triterpenoid, is an abundant, biologically active secondary metabolite that is found in birch species (*Betula* ssp.) [1]. The amount of betulin from different birch species ranges from more than 15% of dry weight in *B. populifolia* and *B. payrifera* to about 30% in *B. verrucosa*. Betulin is readily extracted from the bark of *Betula* ssp. and is an attractive starting material for making different derivatives, including betulinic acid. Betulinic acid and other betulin derivatives have been shown to exhibit multiple biological activities [2–17]. In addition to the selective oxidation of betulin to produce betulinic acid, other modifications have been carried out at C-3 and C-28 of betulin to make novel compounds for biological testing. Allobetulin (19β,28-Epoxy-18α-olean-3β-ol), (Scheme 1), is one of the compounds that is readily obtained from betulin. Acid-catalyzed rearrangement of betulin produces allobetulin in one step and in good yield, making it a valuable candidate for additional modifications. The ease with which betulin is converted to allobetulin has led to the syntheses of novel compounds that include esters, amines, and glycosides by transforming the 3-OH of allobetulin, along with novel modifications to ring A [18,19]. In our study, allobetulin was obtained from betulin by using hydrogen iodide as a catalyst for the transformation. The hydrogen iodide was generated in solution by the reaction of the primary alcohol on the substrate, betulin, with iodine. The synthesis of 19β,28-Epoxy-18α-olean-3β-ol-2-furoate was accomplished by reacting allobetulin with 2-furoyl chloride in dry dichloromethane.

2. Results and Discussion

Allobetulin was synthesized from betulin by using hydrogen iodide (Scheme 1). The hydrogen iodide was generated in solution by reacting the C-28 hydroxy group of the substrate with iodine. The intermediate produced was R-O-I [Scheme 2]. Protonation of a double bond generated a tertiary carbocation that underwent the Wagner–Meerwein rearrangement.

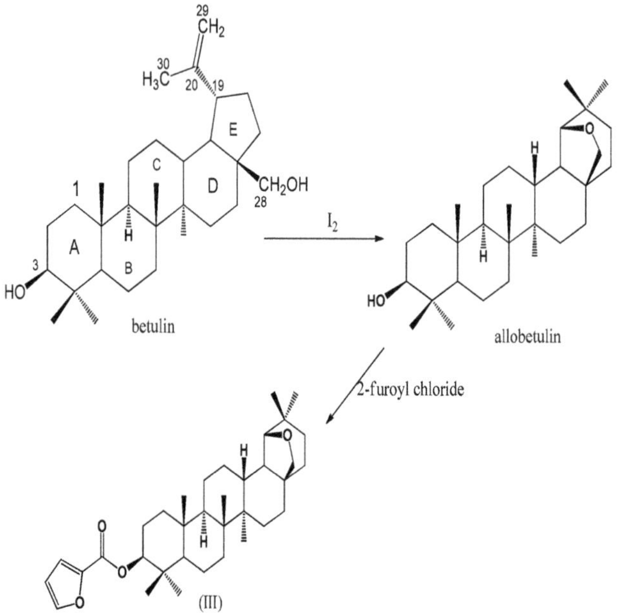

Scheme 1. Synthesis of 19β,28-Epoxy-18α-olean-3β-ol-2-furoate (III).

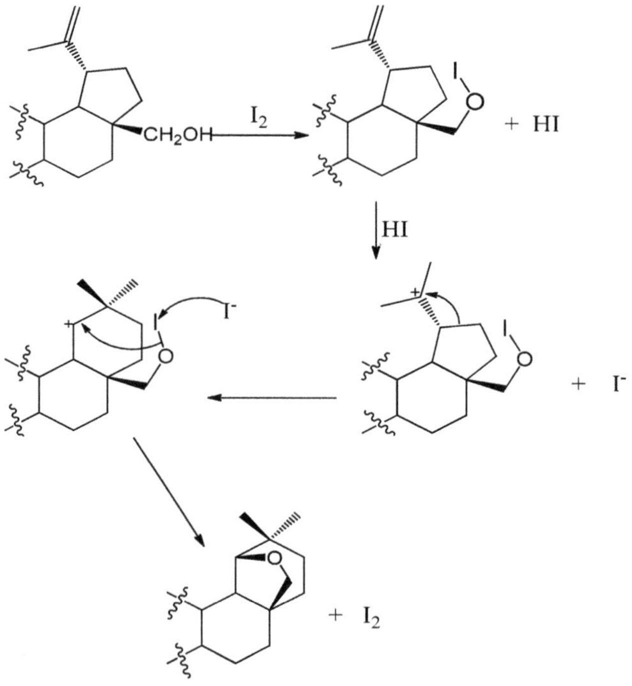

Scheme 2. Hydrogen iodide-catalyzed conversion of betulin to allobetulin.

Green et al. used *p*-toluenesulfonic acid and proposed a mechanism for the rearrangement and cyclization [20]. Recently, Grymel and Adamek used a tetrafluoroboric acid diethyl ether complex to accomplish a similar transformation [21]. The iodide produced during protonation attacks R-O-I, and as the I–I bond is being formed, a new bond develops between oxygen and the carbocation to complete the cyclization. The reaction of iodine with different alcohols has previously been reported [22–24]. The coupling of the first step to the cyclization to produce the final product under mild conditions was not surprising and was in line with past observations. Allobetulin was reacted with 2-furoyl chloride to produce 19β,28-Epoxy-18α-olean-3β-ol-2-furoate (III). The chemical ^{1}H-NMR chemical shifts for most protons did not change much from those of allobetulin. The 3-H_a chemical shift moved from 3.22 ppm to 4.79 ppm because of the ester group at that position. The three additional aromatic protons were centered at 6.51 ppm, 7.15 ppm, and 7.59 ppm, all as doublets of doublets with small coupling constants, in agreement with the findings of Abraham et al. [25] and Bardsley et al. [26]. The ^{13}C-spectra consisted of five new carbons due to the ester -C=O at 158.71, and four aromatic carbons at 111.68 ppm, 117.32 ppm, 145.23 ppm, and 146.13 ppm.

The ^{13}C-DEPT indicated twenty-seven carbon atoms consisting of CH, CH_2 and CH_3 leaving out C1′, C2′ and six quaternary carbons that are part of the triterpene skeleton.

3. Experimental

Betulin was isolated from white birch bark that was collected from York County, Pennsylvania. Dichloromethane, iodine, 2-furoyl chloride, and solvents were purchased from Aldrich. Dichloromethane was dried using molecular sieves (3 Å) that had been activated at 90 °C. ^{1}H and ^{13}C spectra were obtained using a Varian Gemini 500 NMR and recorded at 500 MHz and 125.74 MHz. The spectra are provided as Supplementary Materials. Elemental analysis was performed by Robertson Microlit Laboratories Inc., Legdewood, NJ, USA. Pulverized dry bark (100 g) was suspended in 375 mL of acetic acid: ethyl acetate: ethanol: water (1.5:1:0.5 *v*/*v*). After 48 h at room temperature, the mixture was filtered, and the filtrate was concentrated under vacuum. The solid (17.2 g) was recrystallized from isopropyl alcohol to give pure betulin, m.p. 252–253 °C, (lit. m.p. 254 °C) [27].

3.1. 19β,28-Epoxy-18α-olean-3β-ol (II) (Allobetulin)

To the solution of betulin (0.11 g, 0.034 mmol) in dry dichloromethane (10 mL) molecular sieves (2 g) and iodine (0.04 g, 0.16 mmol) were added. The mixture was stirred at room temperature for 16 h, followed by the addition of a 5% solution of sodium thiosulfate (10 mL). The colorless dichloromethane layer was washed with 5% sodium bicarbonate and then water, dried (Na_2SO_4) and concentrated under vacuum. The solid residue was re-crystallized from ethyl acetate to give the product (0.79 g, 70%) as white flakes, m.p. 258–260 °C, (lit. m.p. 260–261 °C) [28]. ^{1}H-NMR (500 MHz, Me_2SO-d_6) d 0.78 (s, -CH_3), 0.81 (s, -CH_3), 0.86 (s, -CH_3), 0.93 (s, -CH_3), 0.95 (s, -CH_3), 0.99 (s, -2CH_3), 1.25–1.94 (m, -CH_2), 3.22 (dd, J = 5.0 Hz, J = 11.5 Hz, 3-H_a), 3.46 (d, J = 7.5 Hz, H-19), 3.55 (s, 28-H), 3.8 (dd, J = 7.5 Hz, J = 1.5 Hz, H-19). ^{13}C-NMR (125.74 MHz, Me_2SO-d_6) d 13.52, 15.39, 15.72, 16.49, 18.27, 21.00, 24.56, 26.27, 26.45, 26.46, 27.42, 27.99, 28.82, 32.72, 33.92, 34.16, 36.28, 36.76, 37.27, 38.90, 38.93, 40.62, 40.72, 41.49, 46.84, 51.09, 55.50, 71.28 (C-28), 78.97 (C-3), 87.95 (C-19).

3.2. 19β,28-Epoxy-18α-olean-3β-ol-2-furoate (III)

2-Furoyl chloride (0.13 g, 1 mmol) was added dropwise over 5 min to a stirred ice-cold solution of 19β,28-Epoxy-18α-olean-3β-ol (0.22 g, 0.5 mmol) in dry pyridine (4 mL). The reaction mixture was kept at room temperature for 1 h. Ether (20 mL) was added, followed by 5 mL of 1 M HCl solution. The organic layer was washed with 5 % sodium bicarbonate, dried over anhydrous magnesium sulfate, and the ether was removed under vacuum to give a white solid (0.22 g, 84%). Pure crystals were obtained after recrystallization from a mixture of ethyl acetate and hexane (m.p. 300–302 °C). ^{1}H-NMR (500 MHz, Me_2SO-d_6) d 0.82 (s, -CH_3), 0.93 (s, -CH_3), 0.94 (s, -CH_3), 0.95 (s, -CH_3), 0.97 (s, -CH_3), 01.01 (s, -CH_3), 1.26–1.99 (m, -CH_2), 3.46 (d, J = 7.5 Hz, H-28), 3.55 (s, 19-H), 3.80 (d, J = 6.5 Hz, H-28), 4.73 (dd, J = 9.0 Hz, J = 5.5 Hz, 3-H_a), 6.51 (dd, J = 3.5 Hz, J = 1.5 Hz, 1H, aromatic), 7.15 (dd, J = 3.50 Hz, J = 1.0 Hz, 1H, aromatic), 7.594 (dd, J = 1.5 Hz, J = 1.0 Hz, 1H, aromatic). ^{13}C-NMR (125.74 MHz, Me_2SO-d_6) d 13.51, 15.73, 16.58, 16.63, 18.17, 21.04, 23.82, 24.56, 26.27, 26.44, 26.45, 28.02, 28.82, 32.73, 33.86, 34.17, 36.29, 36.76, 37.21, 38.18, 38.60, 40.66, 40.75, 41.50, 46.84, 51.02, 55.59, 71.30, 81.64, 87.98 (-O-C=O), 111.68 (C-aromatic), 117.32 (C-aromatic), 145.23 (C-aromatic), 146.13 (C-aromatic), 158.71 (C=O). $C_{35}H_{52}O_4$ requires: C, 78.31%; H, 9.76%; O, 11.92%. Found: C, 78.29; H, 9.77%, O, 11.95%.

Supplementary Materials: The following supporting information can be downloaded online. Copies of ^{1}H NMR and ^{13}C NMR spectra.

Funding: Funds from the Pennsylvania State University–York Advisory Board were used for this work.

Data Availability Statement: Copies of ^{1}H NMR and ^{13}C NMR spectra.

Conflicts of Interest: The author declares no conflict of interest.

References

1. Krol, S.K.; Kiełbus, M.; Rivero-Müller, A.; Stepulak, A. Comprehensive Review on Betulin as a Potent Anticancer Agent. *BioMed Res. Int.* **2015**, *2015*, 584189. [CrossRef] [PubMed]
2. Sami, A.; Taru, M.; Salme, K.; Jari, Y.-K. Pharmacological properties of the ubiquitous natural product betulin. *Eur. J. Pharm. Sci.* **2006**, *29*, 1–13.
3. Soler, F.; Poujade, C.; Evers, M.; Carry, J.-C.; Hénin, Y.; Bousseau, A.; Huet, T.; Pauwels, R.; De Clercq, E.; Mayaux, J.-F.; et al. Betulinic Acid Derivatives: A New Class of Specific Inhibitors of Human Immunodeficiency Virus Type 1 Entry. *J. Med. Chem.* **1996**, *39*, 1069–1083. [CrossRef] [PubMed]
4. Kashiwada, Y.; Hashimoto, F.; Cosentino, L.M.; Chen, C.-H.; Garrett, P.E.; Lee, K.-H. Betulinic Acid and Dihydrobetulinic Acid Derivatives as Potent Anti-HIV Agents. *J. Med. Chem.* **1996**, *39*, 1016–1017. [CrossRef] [PubMed]
5. Tolstikov, G.A.; Flekhter, O.B.; Shultz, E.E.; Baltina, L.A.; Tolstikov, A.G. Betulin and Its Derivatives. Chemistry and Biological Activity. *Chem. Sustain. Dev.* **2005**, *13*, 1–29.
6. Zhang, D.-M.; Xu, H.-G.; Wang, L.; Li, Y.-J.; Sun, P.-H.; Wu, X.-M.; Wang, G.-J.; Chen, W.-M.; Ye, W.-C. Betulinic Acid and its Derivatives as Potential Antitumor Agents. *Med. Res. Rev.* **2015**, *35*, 1127–1155. [CrossRef]
7. Bori, I.D.; Hung, H.-Y.; Qian, K.; Chen, C.-H.; Morris-Natschke, S.L.; Lee, K.-H. Anti-AIDS agents 88. Anti-HIV conjugates of betulin and betulinic acid with AZT prepared via click chemistry. *Tetrahedron Lett.* **2012**, *53*, 1987–1989. [CrossRef]
8. Hordyjewska, A.; Ostapiuk, A.; Horecka, A.; Kurzepa, J. Betulin and betulinic acid: Triterpenoids derivatives with a powerful biological potential. *Phytochem. Rev.* **2019**, *18*, 929–951. [CrossRef]
9. Kommera, H.; Kaluđerović, G.N.; Kalbitz, J.; Paschke, R. Synthesis and Anticancer Activity of Novel Betulinic acid and Betulin Derivatives. *Arch. Pharm.* **2010**, *343*, 449–457. [CrossRef]
10. Soica, C.M.; Dehelean, C.A.; Peev, C.; Aluas, M.; Zupkó, I.; Kása, P., Jr.; Alexa, E. Physico-chemical comparison of betulinic acid, betulin and birch bark extract and in vitro investigation of their cytotoxic effects towards skin epidermoid carcinoma (A431), breast carcinoma (MCF7) and cervix adenocarcinoma (HeLa) cell lines. *Nat. Prod. Res.* **2012**, *26*, 968–974. [CrossRef]
11. Zhao, J.; Li, R.; Pawlak, A.; Henklewska, M.; Sysak, A.; Wen, L.; Yi, J.E.; Obmińska-Mrukowicz, B. Antitumor Activity of Bet-ulinic Acid and Betulin in Canine Cancer Cell Lines. *In Vivo* **2018**, *32*, 1081–1088. [CrossRef] [PubMed]
12. Tubek, B.; Mituła, P.; Niezgoda, N.; Kempińska, K.; Wietrzyk, J.; Wawrzeńczyk, C. Synthesis and Cytotoxic Activity of New Betulin and Betulinic Acid Esters with Conjugated Linoleic Acid (CLA). *Nat. Prod. Commun.* **2013**, *8*, 435–438. [CrossRef] [PubMed]
13. Shi, W.; Tang, N.; Yan, W.-D. Synthesis and cytotoxicity of triterpenoids derived from betulin and betulinic acid via click chemistry. *J. Asian Nat. Prod. Res.* **2014**, *17*, 159–169. [CrossRef] [PubMed]
14. Kvasnica, M.; Sarek, J.; Klinotova, E.; Dzubak, P.; Hajduch, M. Synthesis of phthalates of betulinic acid and betulin with cytotoxic activity. *Bioorg. Med. Chem.* **2005**, *13*, 3447–3454. [CrossRef] [PubMed]
15. Yamashita, K.; Lu, H.; Lu, J.; Chen, G.; Yokoyama, T.; Sagara, Y.; Manabe, M.; Kodama, H. Effect of three triterpenoids, lupeol, betulin, and betulinic acid on the stimulus-induced superoxide generation and tyrosyl phosphorylation of proteins in human neutrophils. *Clin. Chim. Acta* **2002**, *325*, 91–96. [CrossRef]
16. Gauthier, C.; Legault, J.; Lavoie, S.; Rondeau, S.; Tremblay, S.; Pichette, A. Synthesis and Cytotoxicity of Bidesmosidic Betulin and Betulinic Acid Saponins. *J. Nat. Prod.* **2008**, *72*, 72–81. [CrossRef]

17. Oloyede, H.; Ajiboye, H.; Salawu, M. Influence of oxidative stress on the antibacterial activity of betulin, betulinic acid and ursolic acid. *Microb. Pathog.* **2017**, *111*, 338–344. [CrossRef]
18. Arrous, I.; Boudebouz, O.; Voronova, O.; Plotnikov, E.; Bakibaev, A. Synthesis and antioxidant evaluation of some new allobetulin esters. *Rasayan J. Chem.* **2019**, *12*, 1032–1037. [CrossRef]
19. Dehaen, W.; Mashentseva, A.A.; Seitembetov, T.S. Allobetulin and Its Derivatives: Synthesis and Biological Activity. *Molecules* **2011**, *16*, 2443–2466. [CrossRef]
20. Green, B.; Bentley, M.D.; Chung, B.Y.; Lynch, N.G.; Jensen, B.L. Isolation of Betulin and Rearrangement to Allobetulin. A Biomimetic Natural Product Synthesis. *J. Chem. Educ.* **2007**, *84*, 1985. [CrossRef]
21. Grymel, M.; Adamek, J. Allobetulin. *Molbank* **2022**, *2022*, M1446. [CrossRef]
22. Kasa, A.; Varala, R.; Swami, P.M.; Zubaidha, P. Selective and efficient etherification of secondary cinnamyl alcohols in the presence of iodine catalyst and evaluation of their anti-candida activity. *Chem. J.* **2013**, *03*, 66–74.
23. Kasashima, Y.; Fujimoto, H.; Mino, T.; Sakamoto, M.; Fujita, T. An Efficient Synthesis of Five-membered Cyclic Ethers from 1,3-Diols Using Molecular Iodine as a Catalyst. *J. Oleo Sci.* **2008**, *57*, 437–443. [CrossRef] [PubMed]
24. Kasashima, Y.; Uzawa, A.; Hashimoto, K.; Nishida, T.; Murakami, K.; Mino, T.; Sakamoto, M.; Fujita, T. Synthesis of Cinnamyl Ethers from .ALPHA.-Vinylbenzyl Alcohol Using Iodine as Catalyst. *J. Oleo Sci.* **2010**, *59*, 549–555. [CrossRef] [PubMed]
25. Abraham, R.J.; Bernstein, H.J. The proton resonance spectra of furan and pyrrole. *Can. J. Chem.* **1959**, *37*, 1056–1065. [CrossRef]
26. Bardsley, B.; Smith, M.S.; Gibbon, B.H. Structure elucidation and spectroscopic analysis of photodegradants of the anti-rhinitis drug fluticasone furoate. *Org. Biomol. Chem.* **2010**, *8*, 1876–1880. [CrossRef]
27. Schulze, H.; Pierok, K. Zur Kenntnis des Betulins. *Ber. Dtsch. Chem. Ges.* **1922**, *55*, 2332. [CrossRef]
28. Pettit, G.R.; Green, B.; Bowyer, W.J. Steroids and Related Natural Products. VI. The Structure of α-Apoallobetulin. *J. Org. Chem.* **1961**, *8*, 2879–2883. [CrossRef]

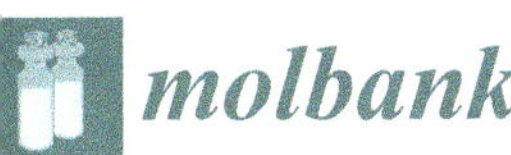 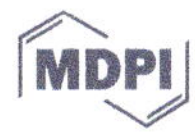

hort Note

3-Methylene-2,3-dihydronaphtho[2,3-*b*][1,4]dioxin-2-yl)methanol

orenzo Suigo †, Giulia Lodigiani †, Valentina Straniero * and Ermanno Valoti

Dipartimento di Scienze Farmaceutiche, Università degli Studi di Milano, Via Luigi Mangiagalli 25, 20133 Milano, Italy
* Correspondence: valentina.straniero@unimi.it; Tel.: +39-02-5031-9361
† These authors contributed equally to this work.

Abstract: (3-Methylene-2,3-dihydronaphtho[2,3-*b*][1,4]dioxin-2-yl)methanol was unexpectedly achieved as the main reaction product while applying a standard Johnson–Corey–Chaykovsky procedure to the 2,3-dihydronaphtho[2,3-*b*][1,4]dioxine-2-carbaldehyde, aiming at obtaining the corresponding epoxide. The structure of the recovered compound was confirmed through NMR and HRMS, the melting point was measured by DSC, and the organic purity was assessed using HPLC. We hypothesized the possible mechanism for the obtainment of this side product, which should involve the opening of the dioxane ring soon after the nucleophilic attack of the ylide to the carbonyl function. The consequent transfer of the negative charge allows the achievement of the phenolate function. The tautomer further rearranges, forming the unstable oxirane, which opening is favored by the acidic phenolic function, thus closing into the more stable six-membered ring compound. We confirmed the hypothesized reaction mechanism by applying the same reaction conditions while starting from the corresponding methyl ketone. This undesired compound, easily and quantitatively obtained by standard Johnson–Corey–Chaykovsky conditions, could pave the way to a new methodology for the obtainment of 2,3-disubstituted 1,4-naphthodioxanes, further derivatizable.

Keywords: 1,4-naphthodioxane; dioxane ring opening; Corey–Chaykovsky epoxidation; Corey–Chaykovsky byproducts

:itation: Suigo, L.; Lodigiani, G.; traniero, V.; Valoti, E. (3-Methylene-,3-dihydronaphtho[2,3-*b*][1,4]dioxin--yl)methanol. *Molbank* **2022**, *2022*, 11521. https://doi.org/10.3390/11521

cademic Editors: Stefano D'Errico nd Annalisa Guaragna

eceived: 17 November 2022
ccepted: 2 December 2022
ublished: 6 December 2022

ublisher's Note: MDPI stays neutral vith regard to jurisdictional claims in ublished maps and institutional affil-ations.

1. Introduction

The Johnson–Corey–Chaykovsky reaction, which is often simplified to Corey–Chaykovsky reaction, is an important tool in organic chemistry to convert alkenes, imines, and aldehydes or ketones to cyclopropanes, aziridines, and epoxides, respectively, while adding one carbon atom to the system through the treatment with sulfur ylides [1,2]. Often, these ylides are in situ formed by treating the corresponding sulfonium (or sulfoxonium) salt with strong bases. The most exploited application of the Corey–Chaykovsky reaction is the direct obtainment of epoxides from aldehydes and ketones, with plenty of examples reported in the literature [3,4]. The reaction mechanism involves the initial nucleophilic attack of the sulfur ylide to the carbonyl of the aldehyde/ketone. Then, the so-formed intermediate undergoes ring closure via intramolecular nucleophilic substitution due to the good leaving nature of the sulfonium group [5].

Although Corey–Chaykovsky reactions usually evolve to the desired products, several other chemical transformations could occur. For instance, the excess of base and high temperatures were reported to promote Yurchenko diolefination of cyclic ketones while suppressing oxirane formation [6]. Moreover, Wang and collaborators disclosed the conversion of esters to α-chloroketones through a reaction with dimethylsulfoxonium methylide in mild conditions, followed by treatment with HCl [7]. Besides these few cases, the Corey–Chaykovsky reaction is considered a very useful and reliable tool for the insertion of an additional carbon atom with ring formation while avoiding dangerous reactants such as diazomethane.

While developing novel antimicrobials, we recently obtained promising compounds as FtsZ inhibitors [8] with a naphthodioxane benzamide structure (Figure 1). Since these derivatives are characterized by an ethylenoxy linker, which could be additionally derivatized through the insertion of specific groups, we decided to apply the Corey–Chaykovsky reaction to achieve a common epoxydic intermediate (**2**). Compound **2** could be easily further converted into the desired compounds by ring opening (Figure 1), thus obtaining a sub-family of compounds with interesting and exploitable features.

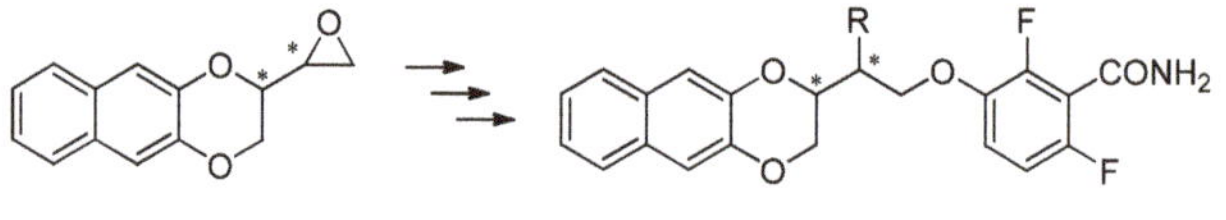

Figure 1. Structure of the epoxydic intermediate **2**, starting material for the obtainment of naphthodioxane benzamide derivatives as FtsZ inhibitors (* no defined chiral center).

For the obtainment of compound **2**, following what was previously performed on the benzodioxane derivatives [9], we designed and applied a straightforward synthetic pathway starting from naphtalen-2,3-diol, where the last step was the Corey–Chaykovsky epoxidation of the corresponding aldehyde (Scheme 1). In the present work, we report the completely unexpected evolution of the Corey–Chaykovsky reaction, leading to an unsaturated alcoholic derivative **1** with good yields and as the main outcome of the reaction. The unknown compound was exhaustively characterized, and the reaction mechanism responsible for its formation was first hypothesized and later confirmed.

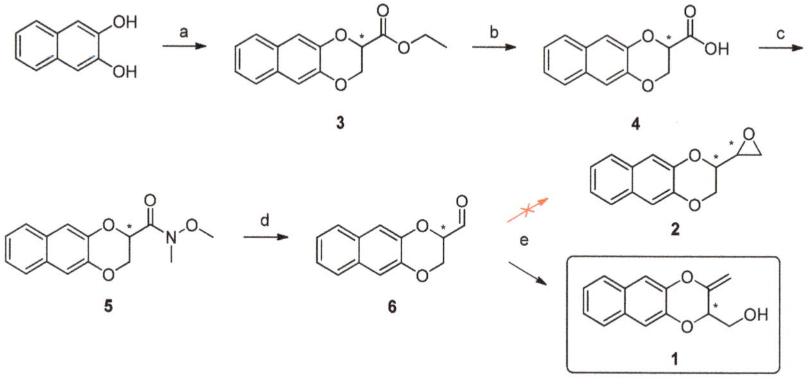

Scheme 1. Synthetic pathway designed for the obtainment of compound **2**; as pointed out, also from the crossed out red arrow, the last reaction failed to give the desired epoxide **2**. Reagents and conditions: (a) Ethyl 2,3-dibromopropionate, K_2CO_3, DMF, 80 °C, 4 h; (b) 2.5 N aqueous NaOH MeOH, RT, 18 h; (c) *N,O*-dimethylhydroxylamine, 1,1′-Carbonyldiimidazole, DMF, RT, 2 h; (d) $LiAlH_4$, THF, −20 °C, 30 min; (e) NaH, trimethylsulfoxonium iodide, DMSO, RT, 30 min. (* no defined chiral center).

2. Results and Discussion

The synthetic scheme (Scheme 1) for the obtainment of compound **2** was designed considering our previous work on benzodioxane benzamides as antibacterial agents [10,11] and other described procedures on benzodioxanes [12] and naphthodioxanes [13–15]. The route started from the reaction between the commercially available naphthalen-2,3-diol with the ethyl 2,3-dibromopropionate in basic conditions, thus achieving the naphthodioxane ring (**3**). We used DMF as a solvent, differently from what was previously reported [13,14], to enhance the conversion and let the obtainment of the ester **3** without any further purification by flash chromatography on silica gel. This ester intermediate underwent hydrolysis (**4**), using milder conditions than previously performed [15], and subsequent conversion to the corresponding Weinreb amide (**5**). Then, the aldehyde was quantitatively achieved by treatment with $LiAlH_4$ at low temperatures (**6**).

By aiming at the obtainment of **2**, **6** was added to a mixture of trimethylsulfoxonium iodide and NaH in dry DMSO. Surprisingly, immediately after the addition of **6** to the in situ formed ylide, the complete conversion of the starting material to the main reaction product was observable through TLC. After the work-up with water and brine and the purification on silica gel, the ^{1}H-NMR spectrum in $CDCl_3$ of the crude revealed the presence of a completely unexpected product, not presenting the classical and diagnostic epoxide signals in the 3 ppm range. On the contrary, four different signals were found in the 3.70–5 ppm range: two coupled doublets with a very tight coupling constant (1.5 Hz) at 4.90 and 4.48 ppm, a double of doublets at 4.69 ppm and a wide signal with an ABX pattern at 3.92–4.00 ppm.

These peculiar NMR chemical shifts and multiplicities, very similar to a 1,4-benzodioxane derivative previously described and obtained following a Pd-catalyzed reaction [16], suggested us to have achieved derivative **1**, and our hypothesis was further confirmed by ^{13}C-NMR and HRMS.

Since compound **1**, differently from **6** and **2**, is substituted not only in the 2-position but also in the 3-positions, this large structural difference moved us to hypothesize a mechanism of the reaction, in which the opening and the re-closing of the 1,4-naphthodioxane ring must occur (Scheme 2).

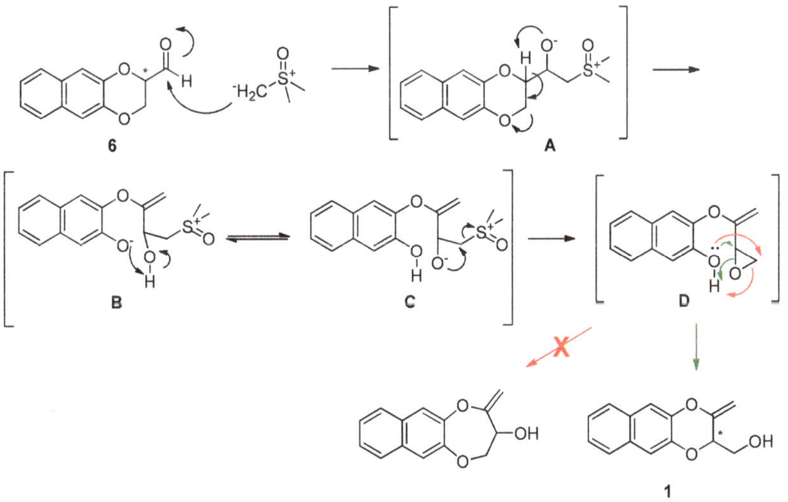

Scheme 2. Proposed mechanism for the obtainment of **1** (* no defined chiral center). Green arrows highlight the observed outcome of the reaction, achieving compound **1**, whereas red arrows indicate the obtainment of a second possible byproduct, which was not achieved in these conditions.

As shown in Scheme 2, our proposed mechanism involves the initial nucleophilic attack of the ylide to the carbonyl, as also expected for the correct evolution of the Corey–Chaykovsky reaction. Nonetheless, in this case, the so formed alcoholate (**A**) does not proceed through the elimination of the sulfonium cation, giving the desired product. Instead, the presence of the two oxygens of the naphthodioxane ring should be responsible for the first deprotonation of the carbon in position 2-, the consequent formation of the unsaturation, the opening of the 1,4-dioxane ring, and the final formation of the phenate function (**B**).

The prototropic equilibrium (**B**,**C**) of this compound could promote the elimination of the sulfonium group by the alcoholate, achieving the epoxide ring (**D**). Subsequently, the acidity of the phenolic function could foster the nucleophilic opening of the oxirane ring, leading to the observed product **1**. In our opinion, both the direct elimination of the sulfonium group by the phenolic function and the oxirane ring opening on the less substituted carbon might be disfavored due to the higher ring strain of the 7-membered ring in such a manner obtained.

We decided to further confirm our hypothetical reaction mechanism by conducting the reaction with a different starting material, the corresponding methyl ketone **7**. The methyl ketone **7** is characterized by the presence of an additional methyl group and could be easily achieved by treating Weinreb amide **5** with methylmagnesium bromide, as previously performed for the benzodioxane derivative [9] (Figure 2). Following our idea, the resulting derivative should be lacking the double of doublets at 4.56 ppm while showing a simplified system at the 3.60–3.96 ppm range and an additional methyl singlet around 1.6 ppm.

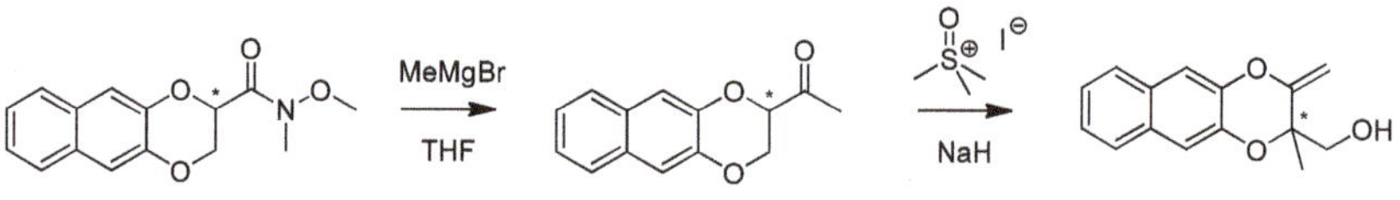

MeMgBr THF NaH 5 7 8

Figure 2. Structure of **8**, obtained as the main product while treating **7** with dimethylsulfoxonium methylide in DMSO at RT (* no defined chiral center).

As expected, the ^{1}H-NMR spectrum of the reaction mixture revealed the achievement of **8** as the main product (Figure 2), even if the TLC and ^{1}H-NMR of the crude showed the presence of other minor byproducts. Nevertheless, also for this derivative, very few traces of the Corey–Chaykovsky epoxide products were observed. The obtainment of **8** further strengthened the hypothesized mechanism presented in Scheme 2.

3. Materials and Methods

All the reagents and solvents were purchased from commercial suppliers (Merck, Darmstadt, DE, Fluorochem, Hadfield, UK, and TCI Europe N.V., Zwijndrecht, BE) and used without any further purifications. Silica gel matrix, with fluorescent indicator 254 nm, was used in analytical thin-layer chromatography (TLC on aluminum foils), and silica gel (particle size 40–63 µm, Merck) was used in flash chromatography on Sepachrom Puriflash XS 420. Visualizations were accomplished with UV light (λ 254 or 280 nm).

The ^{1}H-NMR spectra were measured by Varian Mercury 300 NMR spectrometer/Oxford Narrow Bore superconducting magnet operating at 300 MHz. The ^{13}C-NMR spectra were acquired operating at 75 MHz. Chemical shifts (δ) are reported in ppm relative to residual solvent as the internal standard. Signal multiplicity is used according to the following abbreviations: s = singlet, d = doublet, dd = doublet of doublets, t = triplet, m = multiplet, and bs = broad singlet.

Melting points were measured with a TA Q20 DSC system. IR spectra were recorded with an FT-IR Spectrum TwoTM Perkin Elmer Spectrometer.

The final product **1** was analyzed by reverse-phase HPLC using a Waters XBridge C-18 column (5 µm, 4.6 mm × 150 mm) on an Elite LaChrom HPLC system with a diode array detector (Hitachi, San Jose, CA; USA). Mobile phase: A: H_2O; B: Acetonitrile; gradient, 90% A to 10% A in 25 min with 35 min run time and a flow rate of 1 mL/min. The purity was quantified at their λ max, and the relative retention time is reported in the experimental section. High-resolution mass spectrometry (HRMS) spectra were acquired on Q-Tof SYNAPT G2-Si HDMS 8K (Waters) coupled with an electrospray ionization (ESI) source in positive (ES+) ion mode. The complete characterization of **1** and **8**, in terms of NMR (both ^{1}H and ^{13}C), HPLC, HRMS and IR spectra, are reported in the Supplementary Material.

Ethyl 2,3-dihydronaphtho[2,3-*b*][1,4]dioxine-2-carboxylate (3): A solution of 2,3-di hydroxynaftalene (5.0 g, 31.21 mmol) in DMF (50 mL) was added of potassium carbonate (10.35 g, 74.90 mmol). The reaction mixture was kept stirring at room temperature for 30 min, then ethyl 2,3-dibromopropionate (8.92 g, 34.33 mmol) was added dropwise, and the medium was heated at 80 °C. The reaction mixture was kept stirring at that temperature for 4 h. At reaction completion, the DMF was evaporated, the crude was diluted with ethyl acetate (50 mL) and washed with 10% aqueous NaCl (5 × 20 mL), dried over Na_2SO_4, filtered, and concentrated to give 6.16 g of **3** as an orange oil. Yield: 76%. **^{1}H NMR (300 MHz, $CDCl_3$):** 7.78–7.53 (m, 2H), 7.41 (s, 1H), 7.36–7.29 (m, 2H), 7.28 (s, 1H), 4.92 (dd, *J* = 4.4, 3.1 Hz, 1H), 4.51 (dd, *J* = 11.5, 4.4 Hz, 1H), 4.45 (dd, *J* = 11.5, 4.4 Hz, 1H), 4.28 (q, *J* = 7.1 Hz, 2H), 1.29 (t, *J* = 7.1 Hz, 3H).

2,3-Dihydronaphtho[2,3-*b*][1,4]dioxine-2-carboxylic acid (4): A solution of **3** (6.16 g, 23.85 mmol) in methanol (60 mL) was slowly added of 18 mL of 2.5 N aqueous NaOH. The reaction mixture was kept stirring at room temperature for 18 h. Once the reaction was completed, the methanol was evaporated, and the crude was diluted with ethyl acetate (50 mL) and washed firstly with 10% aqueous HCl (20 mL) and then with 10% aqueous NaCl (20 mL). The organic phase was dried over Na_2SO_4, filtered, and concentrated to give 5.29 g of **4** as a brownish solid. Mp: 187 °C. Mp from the literature [15]: 186 °C. Yield: 96%. **^{1}H NMR (300 MHz, $CDCl_3$):** 7.66 (dd, *J* = 9.3, 4.9 Hz, 2H), 7.40 (s, 1H), 7.32 (dd, *J* = 6.3, 3.2 Hz, 2H), 7.29 (s, 1H), 4.98 (dd, *J* = 4.4, 3.0 Hz, 1H), 4.54 (dd, *J* = 11.6, 4.4 Hz, 1H), 4.47 (dd, *J* = 11.6, 3.0 Hz, 1H).

***N*-Methoxy-*N*-methyl-2,3-dihydronaphtho[2,3-*b*][1,4]dioxine-2-carboxamide (5):** 1,1′-Carbonyldiimidazole (5.58 g, 34.46 mmol) was added portion-wise to a solution of **4** (5.29 g, 22.97 mmol) in DMF (50 mL) at 0 °C. The reaction mixture was stirred at that temperature for 30 min, and then *N*,*O*-dimethyl hydroxylamine hydrochloride (3.36 g, 34.46 mmol) was added to one pot. The mixture was stirred at room temperature for 2 h, and then the volatile components were evaporated. The crude was resumed with ethyl acetate (50 mL), washed with 10% aqueous NaCl (3 × 20 mL), dried over Na_2SO_4, filtered, and concentrated under vacuum to yield 6.26 g of **5** as a yellowish solid. Mp: 119 °C. Yield: 98%. **^{1}H NMR (300 MHz, $CDCl_3$):** 7.65 (dd, *J* = 9.3, 4.9 Hz, 2H), 7.38 (s, 1H), 7.30 (dd, *J* = 6.4, 3.4 Hz, 2H), 7.29 (s, 1H), 5.16 (dd, *J* = 6.5, 2.8 Hz, 1H), 4.50 (dd, *J* = 11.5, 2.8 Hz, 1H), 4.39 (dd, *J* = 11.5, 6.5 Hz, 1H), 3.81 (s, 3H), 3.27 (s, 3H).

2,3-Dihydronaphtho[2,3-*b*][1,4]dioxine-2-carbaldehyde (6): A solution of **5** (1.00 g, 3.66 mmol) in dry THF (15 mL) was added dropwise to a suspension of $LiAlH_4$ (0.18 g, 4.75 mmol) in dry THF (5 mL) at −20 °C under N_2 atmosphere. The reaction mixture was stirred at that temperature for 30 min, then diluted with DCM (15 mL), and coldly washed with 10% aqueous HCl (20 mL) and 10% aqueous NaCl (20 mL). The organic phase was then dried over Na_2SO_4, filtered, and partially concentrated to give 7.8 mL of yellowish crude. Since the aldehyde quickly degrades at room temperature when neat (aldehyde is itself a yellowish oil), a 10% solution in THF was directly used in the successive reaction. **^{1}H NMR (300 MHz, $CDCl_3$)**: 9.84 (s, 1H), 7.65 (m, 2H), 7.43 (s, 1H), 7.35 (m, 2H), 7.29 (s, 1H), 4.74 (t, *J* = 4.2 Hz, 1H), 4.44 (d, *J* = 4.2, 2H).

(3-Methylene-2,3-dihydronaphtho[2,3-*b*][1,4]dioxin-2-yl)methanol (1): A solution of trimethylsulfoxonium iodide (0.93 g, 4.21 mmol) in dry DMSO (10 mL) was added dropwise to a suspension of NaH (0.115 g, 4.40 mmol) in dry DMSO (5 mL) at RT under N_2 atmosphere. After 30 min stirring at that temperature, a solution of **6** (3.66 mmol, 0.78 g, hypothesizing quantitative yield in the previous step) in dry DMSO and THF (3 mL of DMSO and around 7.8 mL of the 10% THF solution coming from the previous step) was added dropwise. The reaction mixture was kept stirring for 1 h at RT and then diluted with Et_2O/AcOEt 9/1 (15 mL) and washed with 10% aqueous NaCl (20 mL) and water (4 × 20 mL). The organic phase was then dried over Na_2SO_4, filtered, and concentrated to give a residue that was purified by flash chromatography. Elution with 85/15 cyclohexane/ethyl acetate gave 0.25 g of **1** as a white solid. Yield: 30% (two steps yield). Mp 100 °C. **^{1}H NMR (300 MHz, $CDCl_3$):** 7.71–7.66 (m, 2H), 7.37–7.33 (m, 4H), 4.90 (d, *J* = 1.5 Hz, 1H),

4.69 (dd, J = 6.8, 5.2 Hz, 1H), 4.48 (d, J = 1.5 Hz, 1H), 3.97 (dd, J = 11.7, 6.8 Hz, 1H), 3.7 (d, J = 11.7, 5.2 Hz, 1H), 2.08 (bs, 1H). **^{1}H NMR (300 MHz, DMSO-d_6):** 7.79–7.69 (m, 2H) 7.45 (s, 1H), 7.41 (s, 1H), 7.37–7.29 (m, 2H), 5.17 (t, J = 5.7 Hz, 1H), 4.83 (d, J = 2.0 Hz, 1H) 4.73 (t, J = 5.7 Hz, 1H), 4.63 (d, J = 2.0 Hz, 1H), 3.68 (t, J = 5.7 Hz, 2H). **^{13}C NMR (75 MHz DMSO-d_6):** 150.5, 142.4, 142.3, 129.9, 129.7, 127.0, 126.8, 125.2, 125.1, 113.1, 111.6, 93.0, 74.3 61.1. HPLC: Purity = 98.3%, T_r = 16.8 min. HRMS (TOF ES+, Na+-adduct): *m/z* 251.0695 252.0728. Calculated mass 251.0684, evaluated mass 251.0695.

1-(2,3-Dihydronaphtho[2,3-*b*][1,4]dioxin-2-yl)ethanone (7): Methylmagnesium bro mide 3.0 M in diethyl ether (5.9 mL) was added dropwise to a solution of **5** (3.23 g 11.82 mmol) in dry THF (45 mL) at 0 °C under N_2 atmosphere. The mixture was stirred a that temperature for 15 min and then warmed to RT and kept stirring for 1 h. After tha timing, it was slowly poured into 10% aqueous HCl (40 mL) and ethyl acetate (40 mL) at (°C. The organic layer was washed with 10% aqueous NaCl (40 mL), dried over Na_2SO_4 filtered, and concentrated under vacuum to yield 2.66 g of **7** as a colorless oil. Yield: 99% **^{1}H NMR (300 MHz, CDCl$_3$):** 7.71–7.64 (m, 2H), 7.41 (s, 1H), 7.33 (m, 2H), 7.29 (s, 1H), 4.7 (dd, J = 5.0, 3.5 Hz, 1H), 4.44 (dd, J = 10.2, 5.0 Hz, 1H), 4.39 (dd, J = 10.2, 3.5 Hz, 1H), 2.34 (s 3H).

(2-Methyl-3-methylene-2,3-dihydronaphtho[2,3-*b*][1,4]dioxin-2-yl)methanol (8): A solution of trimethylsulfoxonium iodide (1.60 g, 7.55 mmol) in dry DMSO (25 mL) was added dropwise to a suspension of NaH (0.20 g, 7.88 mmol) in dry DMSO (15 mL) at RT under N_2 atmosphere. After 30 min stirring at that temperature, a solution of **7** (1.50 g 6.57 mmol) in dry DMSO (10 mL) was added dropwise. The reaction mixture was kept stirring for 1 h at RT and then diluted with Et_2O/AcOEt 9/1 (100 mL) and washed with 10% aqueous NaCl (50 mL) and water (4 × 50 mL). The organic phase was then dried over Na_2SO_4, filtered, and concentrated to give a residue that was purified by flash chromatog raphy. Elution with 80/20 cyclohexane/ethyl acetate gave 0.24 g of **8** as a yellowish solid M.p. 91 °C. Yield: 15%. **^{1}H NMR (300 MHz, CDCl$_3$):** 7.71–7.64 (m, 2H), 7.37–7.31 (m, 4H) 4.90 (d, J = 2.4 Hz, 1H), 4.55 (d, J = 2.4 Hz, 1H), 3.87 (d, J = 11.9 Hz, 1H), 3.71 (d, J = 11.9 Hz 1H), 1.93 (bs, 1H), 1.58 (s, 3H). **^{1}H NMR (300 MHz, DMSO-d_6):** 7.72 (dt, J = 17.9, 6.6 Hz 2H), 7.43 (s, 1H), 7.36 (s, 1H), 7.34–7.29 (m, 2H), 5.22 (t, J = 5.9 Hz, 1H), 4.83 (d, J = 2.2 Hz 1H), 4.66 (d, J = 2.2 Hz, 1H), 3.56 (dd, J = 9.9, 4.5 Hz, 1H), 3.51 (dd, J = 9.9, 4.5 Hz, 1H), 1.48 (s, 3H). **^{13}C NMR (75 MHz, DMSO-d_6):** 154.2, 142.2, 142.1, 130.1, 129.6, 127.0, 126.8, 125.0 124.8, 113.0, 111.1, 92.5, 76.6, 64.7, 21.2. HPLC: Purity= 94.5%, T_r = 10.0 min. HRMS (TOF ES+, Na+-adduct): *m/z* 265.0847, 266.0881, 267.0639, 267.0978. Calculated mass 265.0841 evaluated mass 265.0847.

4. Conclusions

The title compound, (3-methylene-2,3-dihydronaphtho[2,3-*b*][1,4]dioxin-2-yl)methanol was obtained as the main reaction product and with good yields, treating the 2,3-dih ydronaphtho[2,3-*b*][1,4]dioxine-2-carbaldehyde with trimethylsulfoxonium iodide, following the common reaction conditions used in the Johnson–Corey–Chaykovsky reaction. Only negligible traces of the desired corresponding epoxide were found in the reaction mixture The mechanism behind the formation of this side product was firstly hypothesized and then confirmed by applying the same synthetic protocol starting from the analogous methyl ke tone. The (3-methylene-2,3-dihydronaphtho[2,3-*b*][1,4]dioxin-2-yl)methanol, as well as the (2-methyl-3-methylene-2,3-dihydronaphtho[2,3-*b*][1,4]dioxin-2-yl)methanol, were completely characterized by NMR (both ^{1}H and ^{13}C), HPLC, DSC and HRMS. This undesired product could be indeed very useful as a starting material since it bears two differently functionalizable substituents on the 1,4-naphthodioxane ring, not easily achievable via other methods.

Supplementary Materials: The following are available online: Compound **1**; Figure S1: copy of ^{1}H-NMR spectrum in $CDCl_3$; Figure S2: copy of ^{1}H-NMR spectrum in DMSO-d_6; Figure S3: copy of ^{13}C-NMR spectrum in DMSO-d_6; Figure S4: copy of HPLC chromatogram; Figure S5: copy of HRMS spectrum; Figure S6: copy of Elemental Composition Report; Figure S7: copy of IR spectrum; Compound **8**; Figure S8: copy of ^{1}H-NMR spectrum in $CDCl_3$; Figure S9: copy of ^{1}H-NMR spectrum in DMSO-d_6; Figure S10: copy of ^{13}C-NMR spectrum in DMSO-d_6; Figure S11: copy of HPLC chromatogram; Figure S12: copy of HRMS spectrum; Figure S13: copy of Elemental Composition Report; Figure S14: copy of IR spectrum.

Author Contributions: Conceptualization, L.S., V.S. and E.V.; investigation, L.S. and G.L.; data curation, L.S. and V.S.; writing—original draft preparation, V.S. and L.S.; writing—review and editing, V.S. and E.V.; supervision, V.S. and E.V. All authors have read and agreed to the published version of the manuscript.

Funding: This research received no external funding.

Data Availability Statement: The data presented in this study are available in the Supplementary Materials.

Acknowledgments: Mass spectrometry analyses were performed at the Mass Spectrometry facility of Unitech COSPECT at the University of Milan (Italy). The authors would acknowledge Gabriella Roda and Eleonora Casagni for their help in performing IR analyses and the support of the APC fund of the Department of Pharmaceutical Sciences of the University of Milan.

Conflicts of Interest: Authors declare no conflict of interest.

References

1. Corey, E.J.; Chaykovsky, M. Dimethyloxosulfonium Methylide ($(CH_3)_2SOCH_2$) and Dimethylsulfonium Methylide ($(CH_3)_2SCH_2$). Formation and Application to Organic Synthesis. *J. Am. Chem. Soc.* **1965**, *87*, 1353–1364. [CrossRef]
2. Corey, E.J.; Chaykovsky, M. Dimethylsulfonium Methylide, a Reagent for Selective Oxirane Synthesis from Aldehydes and Ketones. *J. Am. Chem. Soc.* **1962**, *84*, 3782–3783. [CrossRef]
3. Adamovskyi, M.I.; Artamonov, O.S.; Tymtsunik, A.V.; Grygorenko, O.O. The synthesis of a 2-azabicyclo [3.1.0]hexane by rearrangement of a spirocyclic epoxide. *Tetrahedron Lett.* **2014**, *55*, 5970–5972. [CrossRef]
4. Kavanagh, S.A.; Piccinini, A.; Fleming, E.M.; Connon, S.J. Urea derivatives are highly active catalysts for the base-mediated generation of terminal epoxides from aldehydes and trimethylsulfonium iodide. *Org. Biomol. Chem.* **2008**, *6*, 1339–1343. [CrossRef] [PubMed]
5. Li, A.-H.; Dai, L.-X.; Aggarwal, V.K. Asymmetric Ylide Reactions: Epoxidation, Cyclopropanation, Aziridination, Olefination, and Rearrangement. *Chem. Rev.* **1997**, *97*, 2341–2372. [CrossRef] [PubMed]
6. Butova, E.D.; Fokin, A.A.; Schreiner, P.R. Beyond the corey reaction: One-step diolefination of cyclic ketones. *J. Org. Chem.* **2007**, *72*, 5689–5696. [CrossRef] [PubMed]
7. Wang, D.; Schwinden, M.D.; Radesca, L.; Patel, B.; Kronenthal, D.; Huang, M.-H.; Nugent, W.A. One-carbon chain extension of esters to alpha-chloroketones: A safer route without diazomethane. *J. Org. Chem.* **2004**, *69*, 1629–1633. [CrossRef] [PubMed]
8. Straniero, V.; Sebastián-Pérez, V.; Suigo, L.; Margolin, W.; Casiraghi, A.; Hrast, M.; Zanotto, C.; Zdovc, I.; Radaelli, A.; Valoti, E. Computational Design and Development of Benzodioxane-Benzamides as Potent Inhibitors of FtsZ by Exploring the Hydrophobic Subpocket. *Antibiotics* **2021**, *10*, 442. [CrossRef] [PubMed]
9. Straniero, V.; Casiraghi, A.; Fumagalli, L.; Valoti, E. How do reaction conditions affect the enantiopure synthesis of 2-substituted-1,4-benzodioxane derivatives? *Chirality* **2018**, *30*, 943–950. [CrossRef] [PubMed]
10. Straniero, V.; Zanotto, C.; Straniero, L.; Casiraghi, A.; Duga, S.; Radaelli, A.; de Giuli Morghen, C.; Valoti, E. 2,6-Difluorobenzamide Inhibitors of Bacterial Cell Division Protein FtsZ: Design, Synthesis, and Structure-Activity Relationships. *ChemMedChem* **2017**, *12*, 1303–1318. [CrossRef] [PubMed]
11. Straniero, V.; Pallavicini, M.; Chiodini, G.; Zanotto, C.; Volontè, L.; Radaelli, A.; Bolchi, C.; Fumagalli, L.; Sanguinetti, M.; Menchinelli, G.; et al. 3-(Benzodioxan-2-ylmethoxy)-2,6-difluorobenzamides bearing hydrophobic substituents at the 7-position of the benzodioxane nucleus potently inhibit methicillin-resistant Sa and Mtb cell division. *Eur. J. Med. Chem.* **2016**, *120*, 227–243. [CrossRef] [PubMed]
12. Artasensi, A.; Angeli, A.; Lammi, C.; Bollati, C.; Gervasoni, S.; Baron, G.; Matucci, R.; Supuran, C.T.; Vistoli, G.; Fumagalli, L. Discovery of a Potent and Highly Selective Dipeptidyl Peptidase IV and Carbonic Anhydrase Inhibitor as "Antidiabesity" Agents Based on Repurposing and Morphing of WB-4101. *J. Med. Chem.* **2022**, *65*, 13946–13966. [CrossRef] [PubMed]
13. Clavier, S.; Khouili, M.; Bouyssou, P.; Coudert, G. Synthesis of naphtho [2,3-*b*][1,4]dioxin, 2-substituted naphtho [2,3-*b*][1,4]dioxins and 2,3-disubstituted naphtho [2,3-*b*][1,4]dioxins. *Tetrahedron* **2002**, *58*, 1533–1540. [CrossRef]
14. Arrault, A. A Straightforward Synthesis of 1,2-Dihydronaphtho [2,1-b]furans from 2-Naphthols. *Synthesis* **1999**, *1999*, 1241–1245. [CrossRef]

15. Howe, R.; Rao, B.S.; Chodnekar, M.S. Beta-adrenergic blocking agents. VII. 2-(1,4-benzodioxanyl) and 2-chromanyl analogs of pronethalol (2-isopropylamino-1-(2-naphthyl)ethanol). *J. Med. Chem.* **1970**, *13*, 169–176. [CrossRef] [PubMed]
16. Dominczak, N.; Lhoste, P.; Kryczka, B.; Sinou, D. Palladium-catalyzed heteroannulation of catechol with functionalized propargylic carbonates: Influence of the functional group on the regioselectivity of the cyclization. *J. Mol. Catal. A Chem.* **2007**, *264*, 110–118. [CrossRef]

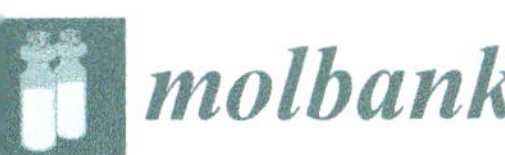

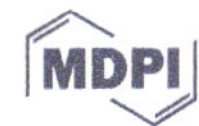

Communication

Obtainment of *Threo* and *Erythro* Isomers of the 6-Fluoro-3-(2,3,6,7,8,9-hexahydronaphtho[2,3-*b*][1,4]dioxin-2-yl)-2,3-dihydrobenzo[*b*][1,4]dioxine-5-carboxamide

Valentina Straniero *, Lorenzo Suigo, Giulia Lodigiani and Ermanno Valoti

Dipartimento di Scienze Farmaceutiche, Università degli Studi di Milano, Via Luigi Mangiagalli, 25, 20133 Milano, Italy

* Correspondence: valentina.straniero@unimi.it; Tel.: +39-02-503-19361

Abstract: 2,6-difluorobenzamides have been deeply investigated as antibacterial drugs in the last few decades. Several 3-substituted-2,6-difluorobenzamides have proved their ability to interfere with the bacterial cell division cycle by inhibiting the protein FtsZ, the key player of the whole process. Recently, we developed a novel family of 1,4-tetrahydronaphthodioxane benzamides, having an ethoxy linker, which reached sub-micromolar MICs towards Gram-positive *Staphylococcus aureus* and *Bacillus subtilis*. A further investigation of their mechanism of action should require the development of a fluorescent probe, and the consequent definition of a synthetic pathway for its obtainment. In the present work, we report the obtainment of an unexpected bicyclic side product, 6-fluoro-3-(2,3,6,7,8,9-hexahydronaphtho[2,3-*b*][1,4]dioxin-2-yl)-2,3-dihydrobenzo[*b*][1,4]dioxine-5-carboxamide, coming from the substitution of one aromatic fluorine by the *in situ* formed alkoxy group, in the final opening of an epoxide intermediate. This side product was similarly achieved, in good yields, by opening the ring of both *erythro* and *threo* epoxides, and the two compounds were fully characterized using HRMS, ^{1}H-NMR, ^{13}C-NMR, HPLC and DSC.

Keywords: 2,6-difluorobenzamide; FtsZ inhibitors; nucleophilic aromatic substitution; side product

Citation: Straniero, V.; Suigo, L.; Lodigiani, G.; Valoti, E. Obtainment of *Threo* and *Erythro* Isomers of the 6-Fluoro-3-(2,3,6,7,8,9-hexahydronaphtho[2,3-*b*][1,4]dioxin-2-yl)-2,3-dihydrobenzo[*b*][1,4]dioxine-5-carboxamide. *Molbank* **2023**, *2023*, M1559. https://doi.org/10.3390/M1559

Academic Editors: Stefano D'Errico and Annalisa Guaragna

Received: 20 December 2022
Revised: 13 January 2023
Accepted: 15 January 2023
Published: 18 January 2023

1. Introduction

The development of novel antibiotics able to modulate innovative targets represents one of the main pursued strategies to fight the worrying problem of antimicrobial resistance [1]. This phenomenon is caused by several human-related factors, such as over-prescription of antibiotics and low investments in the antibiotic resistance field [2].

With the aim of combatting this threat, one of the most exploited and promising bacterial targets is FtsZ (Filamenting temperature sensitive Z) [3], the main protein actor of the bacterial division process, the inhibition of which leads to cell filamentation and lysis [4–7]. Physiologically, GTP-dependent FtsZ polymerization represents the first step of the whole division process, leading to the formation of the Z-ring, a polymeric circular structure, at the site partition. Other division proteins then intervene, forming the mature divisome that allows cytokinesis and cellular division [8].

In the last years, a huge number of FtsZ inhibitors have been developed, belonging to different chemical classes and interacting with the protein on two different binding sites: the GTP-binding site or the Interdomain Cleft (IDC) [4,9–11].

Considering the high variety of FtsZ inhibitors, in terms of chemical structure, origin and interaction site, they are able to inhibit the FtsZ functionality through several mechanisms of actions. For instance, PC190723 (Figure 1), one of the most studied *S. aureus* and *B. subtilis* FtsZ inhibitors, is able to stabilize a high-affinity FtsZ conformation responsible for the assembly, thus exerting antimicrobial activity [12], while other derivatives can interfere with the GTPase activity of FtsZ polymers, evoking again their antimicrobial activity [13].

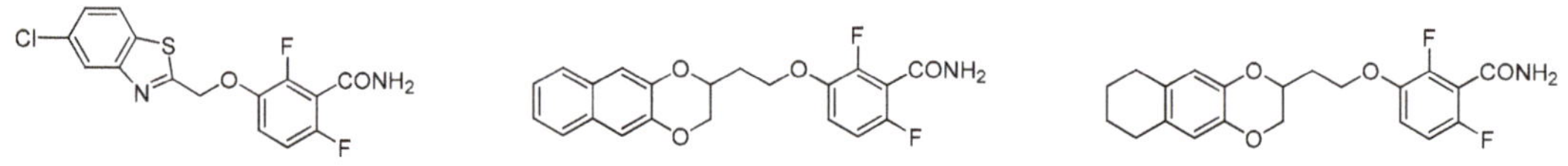

Figure 1. Structures of **PC190723**, derivatives **I** and **II**.

Recently, our research group reported a novel class of 1,4-naphthodioxane- or 1,4-tetrahydronaphthodioxane-benzamides as strong antimicrobials [14], acting through the inhibition of FtsZ, which resulted to be more potent than other benzamides previously reported [5,15–18]. In particular, **I** and **II** (Figure 1) possess MIC values of 0.25 μg/mL and 0.1 μg/mL versus both Methicillin-sensitive and Methicillin-resistant *S. Aureus*, respectively. Moreover, **I** and **II** are both active vs. *B. subtilis* with MICs under 0.1 μg/mL [14].

After having proved their capability to interact and inhibit both *S. aureus* and *B. subtilis* FtsZ, the need of having a fluorescent analogue (Figure 2) of compound **II**, the strongest one, arose. An appropriate probe could indeed help to elucidate FtsZ inhibitors' mechanism of action, as well as to understand any possible off-target interaction, to screen for novel antibiotics, to track antibiotic uptake throughout cells and organisms, and also to detect bacterial infections. Nonetheless, despite the clear and broad utility, the number of fluorescent FZ-probes so far available [19,20] is, to the best of our knowledge, now limited to only a couple of examples.

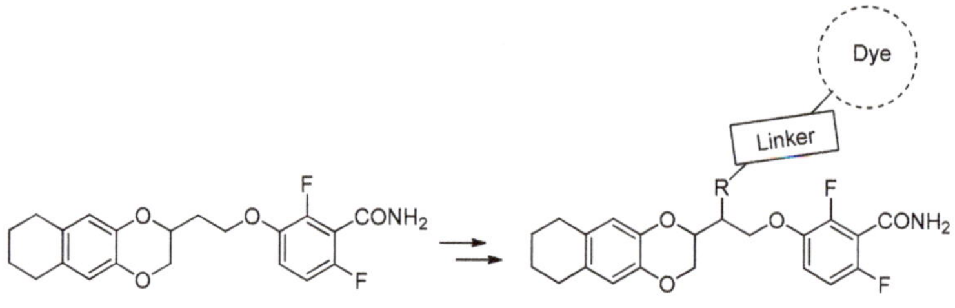

Figure 2. Structures of **II** and of the desired fluorescent analogue.

When thinking how to properly introduce a fluorescent dye, a hydroxylated analogue of **II,** compound **1a**, was designed (Scheme 1), taking inspiration from the work of Stokes and collaborators [21,22]. The introduction of the -OH was intended as a possible anchor point for the binding of a proper linker, and thus a fluorescent dye.

This substituent generates a second stereocenter, and the consequent formation of both *erythro* and *threo* isomers. The obtainment of **1a**, for which we followed Scheme 1, involves the final ring opening of isolated *erythro* and *threo* epoxides. In the present work, we report how both these ring openings could surprisingly allow the achievement, in significant quantities, of the bicyclic side products **1b**, the 6-fluoro-3-(2,3,6,7,8,9-hexahydronaphtho[2,3-*b*][1,4]dioxin-2-yl)-2,3-dihydrobenzo[*b*][1,4]dioxine-5-carboxamides.

We further confirmed how the obtainment of these byproducts **1b** ***erythro*** and ***threo*** is favored during the epoxide opening at quite high temperatures and keeping long reaction times, which are the usual conditions adopted in the final condensation for the preparation of FtsZ inhibitors [14,17,18]. On the contrary, the formation of these side products is partially retarded, keeping milder reaction conditions.

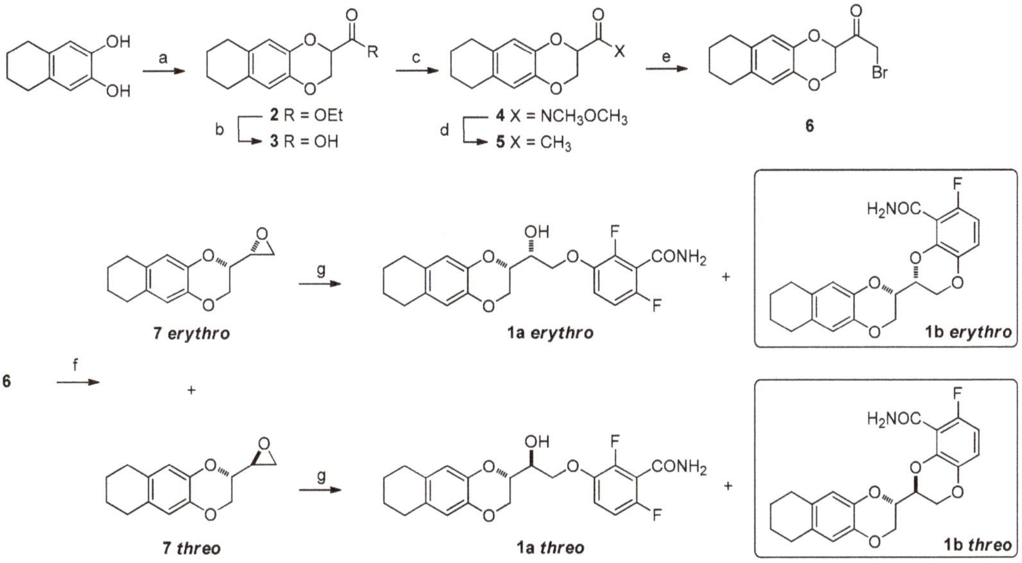

Scheme 1. Synthetic pathway for the obtainment of both **1a** and **1b**. Reagents and conditions: (a) Ethyl 2,3-dibromopropionate, K_2CO_3, DMF, 70 °C, 1 h; (b) 10% aqueous NaOH, MeOH, RT, 30 min; (c) CDI, *N,O*-Dimethyl hydroxylamine hydrochloride, DMF, RT, 2 h; (d) CH_3MgBr, THF, RT, 1.5 h; (e) Br_2, diethyl ether, −5 °C, 3 h; (f) (I) $NaBH_4$, MeOH, 0–5 °C, 30 min; (II) NaH, THF, RT, 18 h; (g) 2,6-difluoro-3-hydroxybenzamide, K_2CO_3, DMF, 70 °C, 18 h.

2. Results and Discussion

The synthetic scheme developed for achieving **1a** is shown in Scheme 1 and started from the 5,6,7,8-tetrahydronaphthalene-2,3-diol, obtained as previously described [14], which was treated with freshly prepared ethyl 2,3-dibromopropionate [23], giving racemic compound **2**. The ester underwent basic hydrolysis, and the resulting carboxylic acid **3** was then converted into the Weinreb amide (**4**). Amide **4** was then quantitatively transformed into the corresponding methyl ketone **5**, by treatment with methylmagnesium bromide, similarly to what was successfully done by our research group on structurally similar derivatives [24,25].

The bromination of methyl ketone **5** was conducted with a single equivalent of bromine at low temperature, to limit the formation of polybrominated side products, and to maximize the conversion into the bromoketone **6**. Then, compound **6** underwent a tandem reaction: the first reduction of the carboxylic function with $NaBH_4$, achieving the instable halohydrin that was soon treated with sodium hydride, affording the two epoxides **7**, both *erythro* and *threo* isomers. The two spots of oxiranes **7** were easily distinguishable through TLC, and the two isomers were thus isolated by flash chromatography on silica gel. Their ^{1}H-NMR spectra in $CDCl_3$ revealed significant differences in terms of chemical shifts and multiplicity (Figure 3).

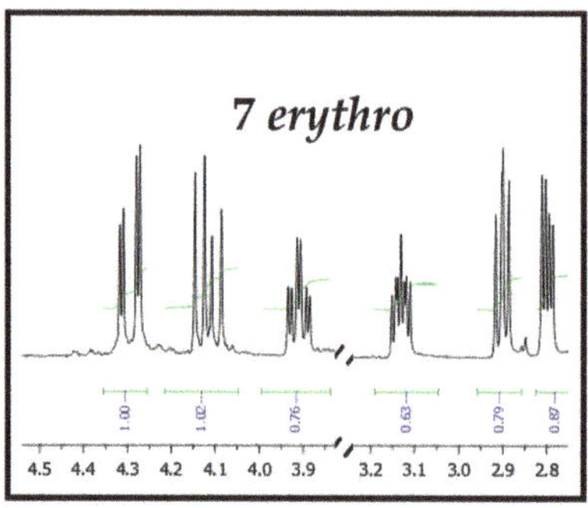

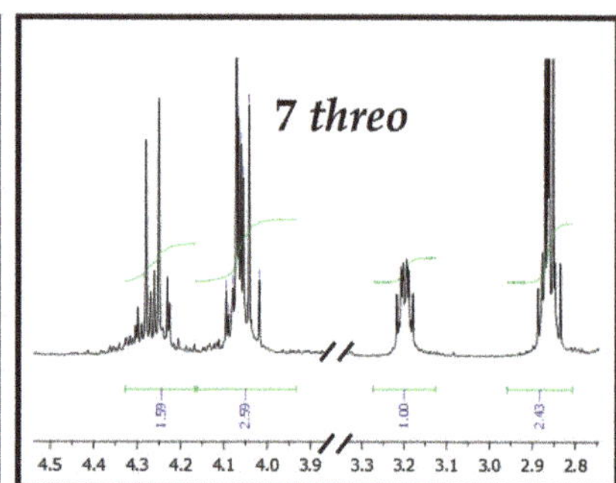

Figure 3. ^{1}H-NMR Spectra extracts of 7 ***erythro*** and 7 ***threo***.

In particular, the first eluted epoxide showed six different signals, with a very clear and defined multiplicity: four doublets of doublets (two at 4.29 and 4.12 ppm, referring to the CH_2 the 1,4-dioxane portion, and two at 2.90 and 2.80 ppm, which are the two hydrogens of the epoxidic CH_2), a doublet of triplets (at 3.91 ppm, diagnostic of the hydrogen of the dioxane CH), and a double of doublets of doublets (3.13 ppm, characteristic for the epoxidic CH). The second eluted oxirane, on the contrary, showed only four multiplets: at 4.26 (1H), 4.07 (2H), 3.19 (1H) and 2.85 (2H) ppm. Moreover, the two appearances were completely different: the first eluted compound was a wax, whereas the second one was a colorless oil. The absence of any literature data on tetrahydronaphthodioxane epoxides moved us to consider the scarce and quite old data on 1,4-dioxane oxiranes [26,27].

Indeed, the peculiar NMR data of the first eluted oxirane were completely in line with what was observed by Clark and coworkers when preparing the enantiopure *erythro*-2-oxiranyl-1,4-benzodioxanes (2*R*, 1′*S*) and (2*S*, 1′*R*). Moreover, also 1,4-benzodioxane *threo* and *erythro* epoxide isomers were strongly different in terms of physic state: enantiopure *erythro* was a solid with a defined melting point (63–64 °C [27]), while the racemic one was defined as oil or with a lower melting point [26,27]. The perfect NMR overlapping, and comparable physical state difference let us define, without doubts, the diastereoisomeric identity of the two epoxides **7**.

The two **7** isomers were parallelly treated at 70 °C for 18 h in basic conditions, in the presence of 2,6-difluoro-3-hydroxybenzamide, to achieve the two final products **1a**. Unexpectedly, the TLC of the two reaction mixtures revealed the presence of two main products, different in terms of chromatographic run. In addition to the one that should refer to the desired compound **1a**, a higher spot was clearly visible in both the reactions, suggesting the formation of a more lipophilic side product.

The two reaction mixtures were worked up and the crudes purified by flash chromatography, letting the isolation, similarly in the two cases, of an undesired compound. Their ^{1}H-NMR spectra showed a surprising pattern for the aromatic signals of the benzamide. We indeed expected to observe the two doublets of triplets, which were diagnostic of the presence of two different fluorine atoms. On the contrary, both the NMR spectra revealed a triplet and a doublet of doublets, suggesting us the absence of one of the two fluorine atoms. Considering the basic reaction conditions and the prolonged reaction times, we hypothesize the formation of the two **1b** side products, in which the epoxide ring opening was soon followed by the *in situ* generation of the alcoholate, and the subsequent benzodioxane ring closure, achieving the bicyclic derivatives **1b *erythro*** and **1b *threo***.

We further confirmed the identity of the two side products by evaluating their ^{13}C-NMR spectra and their HRMS spectra. The presence of six doublets, instead of six doublets of doublets, was indeed the clear sign of the presence of a single fluorine atom. Moreover, the mass analysis confirmed the hypothesis and the elemental compositions.

We also repeated the final steps, by decreasing the reaction temperature or the reaction times, and we noticed how the side products yields were a little lower, further confirming the importance of the reaction conditions.

Finally, we also treated both **1a** ***erythro*** and **1a** ***threo*** while keeping the same reaction conditions used in the ring openings, and we noticed the formation of both **1b** ***erythro*** and **1b** ***threo***, even with low yields.

The partial obtainment of these side products, directly from **1a** ***erythro*** and **1a** ***threo***, suggests how these byproducts are most favored during the epoxides opening. In our opinion, the side products formation could be promoted by a concerted mechanism, in which the ring opening by the phenate is simultaneous to the cyclization due to nucleophilic substitution of the fluorine atom in phenate *ortho* position.

3. Materials and Methods

Starting materials and solvents were purchased from commercial suppliers (Merck, Darmstadt, DE, Fluorochem, Hadfield, UK, and TCI Europe N.V., Zwijndrecht, BE) and were used without further purification.

^{1}H- and ^{13}C-NMR spectra were acquired on a Varian 300 Mercury NMR spectrometer operating at 300 MHz for ^{1}H-NMR, and 75 MHz for ^{13}C-NMR; the chemical shifts are reported in ppm. Signal multiplicity is used according to the following abbreviations: s = singlet, bs = broad singlet, d = doublet, dd = doublet of doublets, ddd = doublet of doublets of doublets, td = triplet of doublets, t = triplet and m = multiplet.

Melting points were measured with a TA Q20 DSC system. TLC were performed on standard analytical silica gel layers (thickness 200 μm; aluminum support silica gel 60 matrix with fluorescent indicator 254 nm, Sigma-Aldrich/Merck KGaA, Darmstadt, Germany). Chromatographic purifications were performed, in normal phase, using flash chromatography on Puriflash XS 420 (Sepachrom, Rho (Milan), Italy), and over different flash chromatography cartridges, filled with Merck high purity grade Silica Gel, 70–230 or 230–400 mesh particle size.

The final side products **1b** ***erythro*** and **1b** ***threo***, as well as the benzamide derivatives **1a** ***erythro*** and **1a** ***threo***, were analyzed by reverse-phase HPLC using a Waters XBridge C-18 column (5 μm, 4.6 mm × 150 mm) on an Elite LaChrom HPLC system with a diode array detector (Hitachi, San Jose, CA; USA). Mobile phase: A: H_2O; B: acetonitrile; gradient, 90% A to 10% A in 25 min with 35 min run time and a flow rate of 1 mL/min. The purity was quantified at their λ max (289 nm) and was found to be >90% for all the compounds, and the relative retention time is reported in the experimental section. High-resolution mass spectrometry (HRMS) spectra were acquired on Q-Tof SYNAPT G2-Si HDMS 8K (Waters) coupled with an electrospray ionization (ESI) source in positive (ES+) ion mode. The characterization spectra of **1b** ***erythro*** and **1b** ***threo***, in terms of NMR (both ^{1}H and ^{13}C) and HRMS, is reported in the Supplementary Material.

Ethyl 2,3,6,7,8,9-hexahydronaphtho[2,3-*b*][1,4]dioxine-2-carboxylate (2): A suspension of 5,6,7,8-tetrahydronaphthalene-2,3-diol (1.50 g, 9.14 mmol) and K_2CO_3 (2.78 g, 20.1 mmol) in DMF (15 mL) was stirred at room temperature for 30 min. Ethyl 2,3-dibromoproprionate (2.61 g, 10.05 mmol) was added dropwise and the reaction mixture was stirred at 70 °C for 1 h, the volatile solvent evaporated under vacuum, the residue diluted with ethyl acetate (20 mL), washed with 10% aqueous NaCl (5 × 15 mL), dried with Na_2SO_4, filtered, and concentrated under vacuum to give 1.86 g (78 %) of **2** as a yellowish oil. ^{1}H-NMR (300 MHz, $CDCl_3$): δ 6.70 (s, 1H), 6.56 (s, 1H), 4.77 (t, *J* = 3.8 Hz, 1H), 4.34 (m, 2H), 4.27 (q, *J* = 7.1 Hz, 2H), 2.67 (m, 4H), 1.75 (m, 4H), and 1.29 (t, *J* = 7.1 Hz, 3H).

2,3,6,7,8,9-Hexahydronaphtho[2,3-*b*][1,4]dioxine-2-carboxylic acid (3): 10% aqueous NaOH (5.7 mL) was added to a solution of **2** (1.86 g, 7.09 mmol) in methanol (20 mL). The reaction mixture was stirred for 30 min at RT, volatile solvents were evaporated, and the residue was diluted with ethyl acetate. The organic layer was washed with 10% aqueous HCl then with brine, dried over Na_2SO_4, then filtered and concentrated under vacuum to yield 1.58 g (95%) of **3** as a yellow oil. ^{1}H-NMR (300 MHz, $CDCl_3$) δ 6.70 (s, 1H), 6.59 (s,

1H), 4.85 (dd, *J* = 5.1, 3.0 Hz, 1H), 4.41 (dd, *J* = 11.0, 5.1 Hz, 1H), 4.34 (dd, *J* = 11.0, 3.0 Hz 1H), 2.66 (m, 4H), and 1.74 (m, 4H).

***N*-Methoxy-*N*-methyl-2,3,6,7,8,9-hexahydronaphtho[2,3-*b*][1,4]dioxine-2-carboxamide (4)** 1,1′-Carbonyldiimidazole (1.64 g, 10.1 mmol) was added to a solution of **3** (1.58 g, 6.74 mmol in DMF (16 mL). After stirring for 30 min, *N*,*O*-dimethyl hydroxylamine hydrochloride (0.99 g, 10 mmol) was added in portions, and the reaction mixture was stirred for 2 h. A completion, the DMF was evaporated, and the crude was diluted with ethyl acetate. The organic phase was washed with 10% aqueous $NaHCO_3$, 10% aqueous HCl and finally with brine and then dried over Na_2SO_4, filtered and concentrated under vacuum to yield 1.76 g (95%) of **4** as a brownish oil. ^{1}H-NMR (300 MHz, $CDCl_3$, δ): δ 6.68 (s, 1H), 6.59 (s, 1H), 5.0 (dd, *J* = 6.7, 2.6 Hz, 1H), 4.37 (dd, *J* = 11.4, 2.6 Hz, 1H), 4.24 (dd, *J* = 11.4, 6.7 Hz, 1H), 3.78 (s 3H), 3.26 (s, 3H), 2.66 (m, 4H), 1.74 (m, 4H).

1-(2,3,6,7,8,9-Hexahydronaphtho[2,3-*b*][1,4]dioxin-2-yl)ethanone (5): 3.0 M Methyl magnesium bromide in diethyl ether (3.2 mL) was added dropwise to a solution of **4** (1.76 g 6.35 mmol) in dry THF (65 mL) at 0 °C under N_2. The reaction mixture was stirred at room temperature for 1.5 h and poured into a 1/1 mixture of ethyl acetate and 10% aqueous HC (50 + 50 mL). The organic phase was then washed twice with 10% aqueous NaCl, dried over Na_2SO_4, filtered and concentrated under vacuum to yield 1.34 g (92%) of **5** as a yellowish oil. ^{1}H-NMR (300 MHz, $CDCl_3$): δ 6.69 (s, 1H), 6.58 (s, 1H), 4.56 (dd, *J* = 4.9, 3.5 Hz, 1H) 4.28 (dd, *J* = 11.4, 3.5 Hz, 1H), 4.25 (dd, *J* = 11.4, 4.9 Hz, 1H), 2.68 (m, 4H), 2.29 (s, 3H), and 1.75 (m, 4H).

2-Bromo-1-(2,3,6,7,8,9-hexahydronaphtho[2,3-*b*][1,4]dioxin-2-yl)ethanone (6): Bromine (0.30 mL, 5.8 mmol) was added dropwise to a solution of **5** (1.34 g, 5.77 mmol) in diethyl ether (40 mL) at −5.0 °C. The mixture was stirred at that temperature for 3 h, washed $Na_2S_2O_5$ (10 mL), dried over Na_2SO_4, filtered and concentrated under vacuum, to obtain 1.80 g of **6** as a yellowish oil (quantitative yield). ^{1}H-NMR (300 MHz, $CDCl_3$): δ 6.72 (s 1H), 6.62 (s, 1H), 4.86 (dd, *J* = 4.7, 3.3 Hz, 1H), 4.40 (m, 2H), 4.33 (d, *J* = 14.0 Hz, 1H), 4.1 (d, *J* = 14.0 Hz, 1H), 2.70 (m, 4H), and 1.76 (m, 4H).

Erythro*- and *Threo*- 2-(Oxiran-2-yl)-2,3,6,7,8,9-hexahydronaphtho[2,3-*b*][1,4]dioxine (7)** $NaBH_4$ (0.11 g, 2.9 mmol) was added in portions to a solution of **6** (1.80 g, 5.77 mmol) in MeOH (36 mL) at 0 °C. The reaction mixture was stirred at 0 °C for 30 min, then volatile solvents were removed under vacuum. The crude was diluted with THF (15 mL) and added dropwise to a suspension of 60% NaH (0.28 g, 6.92 mmol) in THF (5 mL) at 0°C under nitrogen atmosphere. After 30 min, the reaction mixture was warmed to RT and stirred for 18 h, then THF was evaporated, and the crude resumed with ethyl acetate (20 mL and phosphate buffer pH = 7 (15 mL). The organic phase was washed with 10% aqueous NaCl, dried over Na_2SO_4, filtered and concentrated under vacuum to yield 1.40 g of a mixture of **7** isomers as a brown oil. Elution with 9/1 cyclohexane/ethyl acetate on silica gel gave 0.47 g of **7 *erythro (first eluted) as white wax and 0.32 g of **7 *threo*** (second eluted as colorless oil (Cumulative yield of *erythro* and *threo* isomers = 59%).

7 Erythro: ^{1}H-NMR (300 MHz, $CDCl_3$): δ 6.60 (s, 2H), 4.29 (dd, *J* = 11.4, 2.4 Hz, 1H) 4.12 (dd, *J* = 11.4, 6.6 Hz, 1H), 3.91 (td, *J* = 6.6, 2.4 Hz, 1H), 3.13 (ddd, *J* = 6.6, 4.1, 2.6 Hz, 1H) 2.90 (dd, *J* = 4.9, 4.1 Hz, 1H), 2.80 (dd, *J* = 4.9, 2.6 Hz, 1H), 2.67 (m, 4H), and 1.73 (m, 4H).

7 Threo: ^{1}H-NMR (300 MHz, $CDCl_3$): δ 6.63 (s, 1H), 6.58 (s, 1H), 4.26 (m, 1H), 4.07 (m 2H), 3.19 (m, 1H), 2.85 (m, 2H), 2.66 (m, 4H), and 1.74 (m, 4H).

Erythro* 2,6-Difluoro-3-(2-(2,3,6,7,8,9-hexahydronaphtho[2,3-*b*][1,4]dioxin-2-yl)-2 hydroxyethoxy)benzamide (1a *erythro*) and *erythro* 6-Fluoro-3-(2,3,6,7,8,9 hexahydronaphtho[2,3-*b*][1,4]dioxin-2-yl)-2,3-dihydrobenzo[*b*][1,4]dioxine-5-carboxamide (1b *erythro*):** A solution of 3-Hydroxy-2,6-difluorobenzamide (0.37 g, 2.1 mmol) in DMF (3 mL) was added to a solution of **7 *erythro (0.47 g, 2.0 mmol) and K_2CO_3 (0.31 g, 2.2 mmol in DMF (2 mL) at RT. Heating and stirring at 70 °C for 18 h led to the obtainment of the side product **1b *erythro*** in 24% yield. DMF evaporation under vacuum, dilution with ethyl acetate (20 mL), washing with 10% aqueous NaCl (5 × 10 mL), drying over Na_2SO_4 filtering and concentration under vacuum gave a brown residue. Elution with 6/4 to 4/6 cyclohexane/ethyl acetate on silica gel allowed the isolation of 0.32 g (Yield = 39%) of **1a** ***erythro*** and of 0.19 g (Yield = 24%) of **1b** ***erythro*** as white solids.

1a ***erythro:*** HPLC: Tr = 14.9 min. Mp = 155 °C.

^{1}H-NMR (300 MHz, d_6-DMSO): δ 8.10 (s, 1H), 7.81 (s, 1H), 7.24 (dt, *J* = 9.3, 5.3 Hz, 1H), 7.04 (dt, *J* = 9.0, 1.8 Hz, 1H), 6.52 (s, 1H), 6.51 (s, 1H), 5.68 (d, *J* = 5.9 Hz, 1H), 4.32 (d, *J* = 9.5 Hz, 1H), 4.15 (m, 4H), 3.94 (m, 1H), 2.55 (m, 4H), and 1.64 (m, 4H)

^{13}C-NMR (75 MHz, d_6-DMSO): δ 161.8, 152.3 (dd, *J* = 239.3, 6.7 Hz), 148.3 (dd, *J* = 246.8, 8.2 Hz), 143.7 (dd, *J* = 10.5, 3.0 Hz), 143.3, 140.8, 129.9, 129.7, 117.0 (dd, *J* = 24.6, 20.3 Hz), 117.0, 116.9, 116.8, 116.7, 116.0 (dd, *J* = 8.5, 1.7 Hz), 111.3 (dd, *J* = 23.1, 3.0 Hz), 73.1, 71.4, 67.8, 64.9, 28.5, and 23.2.

1b ***erythro*****:** HPLC: Tr = 15.3 min. Mp = 266 °C. HRMS (TOF ES$^+$, Na$^+$-adduct): *m/z* 408.1229, 409.1263, and 410.1289. Calculated mass 408.1218, evaluated mass 408.1229.

^{1}H-NMR (300 MHz, d_6-DMSO): δ 7.91 (s, 1H), 7.63 (s, 1H), 6.92 (d, *J* = 9.0, 5.4 Hz, 1H), 6.73 (t, *J* = 9.0 Hz, 1H), 6.58 (s, 1H), 6.55 (s, 1H), 4.44 (dd, *J* = 11.6, 3.5 Hz, 1H), 4.33–4.28 (m, 4H), 4.17 (dd, *J* = 12.1, 6.5 Hz, 1H), 2.57 (m, 4H), and 1.64 (m, 4H).

^{13}C-NMR (75 MHz, d_6-DMSO): δ 163.4, 153.1 (d, *J* = 237.0 Hz), 141.1, 140.1, 139.7 (d, *J* = 3.0 Hz), 139.5 (d, *J* = 9.0 Hz), 130.24, 130.17, 117.6 (d, *J* = 9.0 Hz), 117.03, 117.01, 116.9 (d, *J* = 27.0 Hz), 108.3 (d, *J* = 25.5 Hz), 70.1, 70.0, 64.3, 63.6, 28.5, and 23.2.

Threo **2,6-Difluoro-3-(2-(2,3,6,7,8,9-hexahydronaphtho[2,3-*b*][1,4]dioxin-2-yl)-2-hydroxyethoxy)benzamide (1a *threo*) and *threo* 6-Fluoro-3-(2,3,6,7,8,9-hexahydronaphtho [1,4]dioxin-2-yl)-2,3-dihydrobenzo[*b*][1,4]dioxine-5-carboxamide (1b *threo*): 1a** and **1b** *threo* were obtained from **7** ***threo*** (0.30 g, 1.3 mmol), following the same procedure of **1a** *erythro* and **1b** *erythro*, achieving 0.16 g (Yield = 31%) of **1a** *threo* and 80 mg (Yield = 16%) of **1b** *threo* as white solids.

1a ***threo***: HPLC Tr = 14.5 min. Mp = 147 °C.

^{1}H-NMR (300 MHz, d_6-DMSO): δ 8.09 (s, 1H), 7.81 (s, 1H), 7.27 (dt, *J* = 9.4, 5.3 Hz, 1H), 7.05 (dt, *J* = 9.0, 1.9 Hz, 1H), 6.53 (s, 1H), 6.52 (s, 1H), 5.49 (d, *J* = 5.8 Hz, 1H), 4.33 (dd, *J* = 11.2, 2.0 Hz, 1H), 4.09 (m, 5H), 2.56 (m, 4H), and 1.64 (m, 4H).

^{13}C-NMR (75 MHz, d_6-DMSO): δ 161.8, 152.3 (dd, *J* = 239.3, 6.7 Hz), 148.3 (dd, *J* = 246.8, 8.2 Hz), 143.7 (dd, *J* = 10.5, 3.0 Hz), 143.3, 140.8, 129.9, 129.7, 117.0 (dd, *J* = 24.6, 20.3 Hz), 117.0, 116.9, 116.8, 116.7, 116.0 (dd, *J* = 8.5, 1.7 Hz), 111.3 (dd, *J* = 23.1, 3.0 Hz), 73.1, 71.4, 67.8, 64.9, 28.5, and 23.2.

1b ***threo***: HPLC Tr = 13.3 min. Mp = 290 °C with decomposition. HRMS (TOF ES+, Na+-adduct): *m/z* 408.1222, 409.1253, and 410.1277. Calculated mass 408.1218, evaluated mass 408.1222.

^{1}H-NMR (300 MHz, d_6-DMSO): δ 7.75 (s, 1H), 7.56 (s, 1H), 6.91 (d, *J* = 8.9, 5.5 Hz, 1H), 6.71 (t, *J* = 8.9 Hz, 1H), 6.55 (s, 1H), 6.52 (s, 1H), 4.48-4.37 (m, 4H), 4.21 (dd, *J* = 11.9, 8.1 Hz, 1H), 4.08 (dd, *J* = 11.9, 8.3 Hz, 1H), 2.56 (m, 4H), and 1.64 (m, 4H).

^{13}C-NMR (75 MHz, d_6-DMSO): δ 163.4, 153.2 (d, *J* = 236.8 Hz), 141.0, 140.8 (d, *J* = 3.0 Hz), 140.4 (d, *J* = 10.1 Hz), 139.7, 130.1, 130.0, 117.61 (d, *J* = 9.0 Hz), 117.59, 117.5, 117.0 (d, *J* = 21.1 Hz), 108.2 (d, *J* = 22.3 Hz), 72.1, 71.7, 64.5, 64.2, 28.5, and 23.2.

Conversion of 1a *erythro* to 1b *erythro*: A solution of **1a** ***erythro*** (0.10 g, 0.25 mmol) in DMF (1 mL) was added to a suspension of K_2CO_3 (0.070 g, 0.50 mmol) in DMF (1 mL) at RT. The mixture was heated at 70 °C and stirred for 18 h, then DMF was evaporated under vacuum. The residue was diluted with ethyl acetate (10 mL), washed with 10% aqueous NaCl (5 × 5 mL), dried over Na_2SO_4, then filtered and concentrated under vacuum, yielding a brown residue. Elution with 1/1 cyclohexane/ethyl acetate on silica gel allowed the isolation of 34 mg (35%) of **1b** ***erythro*** as a white solid.

Conversion of 1a *threo* to 1b *threo*: 1b ***threo*** was obtained from **1a** ***threo*** (0.10 g, 0.25 mmol), following the same procedure seen for **1b** ***erythro***, achieving 29 mg (30%) of **1b** ***threo*** as a white solid.

4. Conclusions

The two *threo* and *erythro* isomers of the 6-fluoro-3-(2,3,6,7,8,9-hexahydronaphtho[2,3-*b*][1,4]dioxin-2-yl)-2,3-dihydrobenzo[*b*][1,4]dioxine-5-carboxamide were obtained as a significant and abundant side product, when opening the two isomers of the 2-(oxiran-2-yl)-2,3,6,7,8,9-hexahydronaphtho[2,3-*b*][1,4]dioxines with a 2,6-difluorophenate, stirring at 70 °C and keeping overnight reaction times.

The structure of these two side products was firstly hypothesized by carefully evaluating the ^{1}H-NMR spectra, which revealed the absence of a fluorine atom, and then confirmed by both ^{13}C-NMR and HRMS spectra. The diastereoisomeric identity was defined after having characterized the isomer nature of the starting epoxides, by NMR comparison with literature enantiopure 1,4-benzodixoane oxiranes. The side products were further characterized by HPLC and DSC, fully detailing these novel and unexpected byproducts.

Supplementary Materials: The following are available online: Compound **1b *erythro***; Figure S1: Copy of ^{1}H-NMR spectrum in DMSO-d_6; Figure S2: Copy of ^{13}C-NMR spectrum in DMSO-d_6; Figure S3: Copy of HRMS spectrum; Figure S4: Copy of Elemental Composition Report; Compound **1b *threo***; Figure S5: Copy of ^{1}H-NMR spectrum in DMSO-d_6; Figure S6: Copy of ^{13}C-NMR spectrum in DMSO-d_6; Figure S7: Copy of HRMS spectrum; and Figure S8: Copy of Elemental Composition Report.

Author Contributions: Conceptualization, L.S., V.S. and E.V.; investigation, L.S. and G.L.; data curation, L.S. and V.S.; writing—original draft preparation, V.S. and L.S.; writing—review and editing, V.S. and E.V.; supervision, V.S. and E.V. All authors have read and agreed to the published version of the manuscript.

Funding: This research received no external funding.

Data Availability Statement: The data presented in this study are available in the Supplementary Materials.

Acknowledgments: Mass spectrometry analyses were performed at the Mass Spectrometry facility of Unitech COSPECT at the University of Milan (Italy). The authors acknowledge the support of the APC central fund of the University of Milan.

Conflicts of Interest: The authors declare no conflict of interest.

Sample Availability: Samples of the compounds are available from the authors.

References

1. World Health Organization. Global Action Plan on Antimicrobial Resistance. 2015. Available online: https://www.who.int/publications/i/item/9789241509763 (accessed on 15 October 2022).
2. World Health Organization. Antibiotic Resistance: Prevention and Control. Available online: https://www.who.int/news-room/fact-sheets/detail/antibiotic-resistance#:~{}:text=Antibiotic%20resistance%20is%20accelerated%20by,poor%20infection%20prevention%20and%20control (accessed on 15 October 2022).
3. Pradhan, P.; Margolin, W.; Beuria, T.K. Targeting the Achilles Heel of FtsZ: The Interdomain Cleft. *Front. Microbiol.* **2021**, *12*, 732796. [CrossRef] [PubMed]
4. Casiraghi, A.; Suigo, L.; Valoti, E.; Straniero, V. Targeting Bacterial Cell Division: A Binding Site-Centered Approach to the Most Promising Inhibitors of the Essential Protein FtsZ. *Antibiotics* **2020**, *9*, 69. [CrossRef] [PubMed]
5. Straniero, V.; Pallavicini, M.; Chiodini, G.; Zanotto, C.; Volontè, L.; Radaelli, A.; Bolchi, C.; Fumagalli, L.; Sanguinetti, M.; Menchinelli, G.; et al. 3-(Benzodioxan-2-ylmethoxy)-2,6-difluorobenzamides bearing hydrophobic substituents at the 7-position of the benzodioxane nucleus potently inhibit methicillin-resistant Sa and Mtb cell division. *Eur. J. Med. Chem.* **2016**, *120*, 227–243. [CrossRef] [PubMed]
6. Adams, D.W.; Wu, L.J.; Czaplewski, L.G.; Errington, J. Multiple effects of benzamide antibiotics on FtsZ function. *Mol. Microbiol.* **2011**, *80*, 68–84. [CrossRef] [PubMed]
7. Adams, D.W.; Wu, L.J.; Errington, J. A benzamide-dependent ftsZ mutant reveals residues crucial for Z-ring assembly. *Mol. Microbiol.* **2016**, *99*, 1028–1042. [CrossRef]
8. Haeusser, D.P.; Margolin, W. Splitsville: Structural and functional insights into the dynamic bacterial Z ring. *Nat. Rev. Microbiol.* **2016**, *14*, 305–319. [CrossRef]
9. Carro, L. Recent Progress in the Development of Small-Molecule FtsZ Inhibitors as Chemical Tools for the Development of Novel Antibiotics. *Antibiotics* **2019**, *8*, 217. [CrossRef]
10. Tripathy, S.; Sahu, S.K. FtsZ inhibitors as a new genera of antibacterial agents. *Bioorg. Chem.* **2019**, *91*, 103169. [CrossRef]

1. Han, H.; Wang, Z.; Li, T.; Da, T.; Mao, R.; Hao, Y.; Yang, N.; Wang, X.; Wang, J. Recent progress of bacterial FtsZ inhibitors with a focus on peptides. *FEBS J.* **2021**, *288*, 1091–1106. [CrossRef]
2. Elsen, N.L.; Lu, J.; Parthasarathy, G.; Reid, J.C.; Sharma, S.; Soisson, S.M.; Lumb, K.J. Mechanism of action of the cell-division inhibitor PC190723: Modulation of FtsZ assembly cooperativity. *J. Am. Chem. Soc.* **2012**, *134*, 12342–12345. [CrossRef]
3. Fang, Z.; Li, Y.; Zheng, Y.; Li, X.; Lu, Y.-J.; Yan, S.-C.; Wong, W.-L.; Chan, K.-F.; Wong, K.-Y.; Sun, N. Antibacterial activity and mechanism of action of a thiophenyl substituted pyrimidine derivative. *RSC Adv.* **2019**, *9*, 10739–10744. [CrossRef]
4. Straniero, V.; Sebastián-Pérez, V.; Suigo, L.; Margolin, W.; Casiraghi, A.; Hrast, M.; Zanotto, C.; Zdovc, I.; Radaelli, A.; Valoti, E. Computational Design and Development of Benzodioxane-Benzamides as Potent Inhibitors of FtsZ by Exploring the Hydrophobic Subpocket. *Antibiotics* **2021**, *10*, 442. [CrossRef]
5. Chiodini, G.; Pallavicini, M.; Zanotto, C.; Bissa, M.; Radaelli, A.; Straniero, V.; Bolchi, C.; Fumagalli, L.; Ruggeri, P.; De Giuli Morghen, C.; et al. Benzodioxane-benzamides as new bacterial cell division inhibitors. *Eur. J. Med. Chem.* **2015**, *89*, 252–265. [CrossRef] [PubMed]
6. Straniero, V.; Zanotto, C.; Straniero, L.; Casiraghi, A.; Duga, S.; Radaelli, A.; De Giuli Morghen, C.; Valoti, E. 2,6-Difluorobenzamide Inhibitors of Bacterial Cell Division Protein FtsZ: Design, Synthesis, and Structure-Activity Relationships. *ChemMedChem* **2017**, *12*, 1303–1318. [CrossRef]
7. Straniero, V.; Sebastián Pérez, V.; Hrast, M.; Zanotto, C.; Casiraghi, A.; Suigo, L.; Zdovc, I.; Radaelli, A.; De Giuli Morghen, C.; Valoti, E. Benzodioxane-benzamides as antibacterial agents: Computational and SAR studies to evaluate the influence of the 7-substitution in FtsZ interaction. *ChemMedChem* **2020**, *2*, 195–209. [CrossRef]
8. Straniero, V.; Suigo, L.; Casiraghi, A.; Sebastián-Pérez, V.; Hrast, M.; Zanotto, C.; Zdovc, I.; De Giuli Morghen, C.; Radaelli, A.; Valoti, E. Benzamide Derivatives Targeting the Cell Division Protein FtsZ: Modifications of the Linker and the Benzodioxane Scaffold and Their Effects on Antimicrobial Activity. *Antibiotics* **2020**, *9*, 160. [CrossRef] [PubMed]
9. Artola, M.; Ruíz-Avila, L.B.; Ramírez-Aportela, E.; Martínez, R.F.; Araujo-Bazán, L.; Vázquez-Villa, H.; Martín-Fontecha, M.; Oliva, M.A.; Martín-Galiano, A.J.; Chacón, P.; et al. The structural assembly switch of cell division protein FtsZ probed with fluorescent allosteric inhibitors. *Chem. Sci.* **2017**, *8*, 1525–1534. [CrossRef] [PubMed]
10. Ferrer-González, E.; Fujita, J.; Yoshizawa, T.; Nelson, J.M.; Pilch, A.J.; Hillman, E.; Ozawa, M.; Kuroda, N.; Al-Tameemi, H.M.; Boyd, J.M.; et al. Structure-Guided Design of a Fluorescent Probe for the Visualization of FtsZ in Clinically Important Gram-Positive and Gram-Negative Bacterial Pathogens. *Sci. Rep.* **2019**, *9*, 20092. [CrossRef] [PubMed]
11. Stokes, N.R.; Baker, N.; Bennett, J.M.; Berry, J.; Collins, I.; Czaplewski, L.G.; Logan, A.; Macdonald, R.; Macleod, L.; Peasley, H.; et al. An improved small-molecule inhibitor of FtsZ with superior in vitro potency, drug-like properties, and in vivo efficacy. *Antimicrob. Agents Chemother.* **2013**, *57*, 317–325. [CrossRef]
12. Stokes, N.R.; Baker, N.; Bennett, J.M.; Chauhan, P.K.; Collins, I.; Davies, D.T.; Gavade, M.; Kumar, D.; Lancett, P.; Macdonald, R.; et al. Design, synthesis and structure-activity relationships of substituted oxazole-benzamide antibacterial inhibitors of FtsZ. *Bioorg. Med. Chem. Lett.* **2014**, *24*, 353–359. [CrossRef]
13. Casiraghi, A.; Valoti, E.; Suigo, L.; Artasensi, A.; Sorvillo, E.; Straniero, V. How Reaction Conditions May Influence the Regioselectivity in the Synthesis of 2,3-Dihydro-1,4-benzoxathiine Derivatives. *J. Org. Chem.* **2018**, *83*, 13217–13227. [CrossRef] [PubMed]
14. Suigo, L.; Lodigiani, G.; Straniero, V.; Valoti, E. (3-Methylene-2,3-dihydronaphtho[2,3-b][1,4]dioxin-2-yl)methanol. *Molbank* **2022**, *2022*, M1521. [CrossRef]
15. Straniero, V.; Casiraghi, A.; Fumagalli, L.; Valoti, E. How do reaction conditions affect the enantiopure synthesis of 2-substituted-1,4-benzodioxane derivatives? *Chirality* **2018**, *30*, 943–950. [CrossRef] [PubMed]
16. Clark, R.D.; Caroon, J.M.; Kluge, A.F.; Repke, D.B.; Roszkowski, A.P.; Strosberg, A.M.; Baker, S.; Bitter, S.M.; Okada, M.D. Synthesis and antihypertensive activity of 4′-substituted spiro4H-3,1-benzoxazine-4,4′-piperidin-2(1H)-ones. *J. Med. Chem.* **1983**, *26*, 657–661. [CrossRef] [PubMed]
17. Clark, R.D.; Kurz, L.J. Synthesis of the Enantiomers of Erythro-2-oxiranyl-1,4-benzodioxan. *Heterocycles* **1985**, *23*, 2005. [CrossRef]

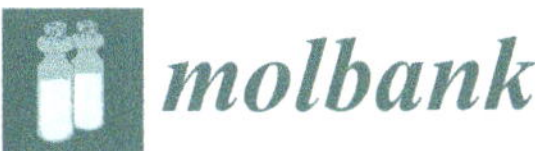 molbank MDPI

Short Note

2-(1-Methoxycarbonyl-2-phenyleth-1-yl)-1-benzylpyridin-1-ium Bromide

Lorenzo Suigo, Valentina Straniero * and Ermanno Valoti

Dipartimento di Scienze Farmaceutiche, Università degli Studi di Milano, Via Luigi Mangiagalli 25, 20133 Milano, Italy; lorenzo.suigo@unimi.it (L.S.); ermanno.valoti@unimi.it (E.V.)
* Correspondence: valentina.straniero@unimi.it; Tel.: +39-02-5031-9361

Abstract: In this work, we report the unexpected conversion of a pyridine derivative into the corresponding *N*-benzylated pyridinium salt due to the presence of unreacted benzyl bromide in the crude product. This transformation was observed at room temperature in a solvent-free environment and without any stirring. These interesting data show how pyridinium salts can be formed in mild conditions, avoiding high temperatures that could promote the degradation of the desired product.

Keywords: quaternary ammonium salts; α-carbon benzylation; *N*-benzylation

1. Introduction

Quaternary ammonium cations are known as versatile functional groups with various applications in many branches of chemistry. Within organic chemistry, ammonium cations are widely present in structures of phase-transfer compounds [1] (for instance, tetrabutylammonium bromide), drugs (neuromuscular-blocking drugs, cholinergic drugs, antimicrobials [2]), surfactants (phosphatidylcholines) and many others. In synthesis, due to their electrophilic nature, quaternary ammonium cations are also exploited as leaving groups in nucleophilic substitutions [3,4]. The most common method of synthesizing quaternary pyridinium or ammonium salts is the Menšutkin reaction, i.e., simple alkylation with alkyl halides, which often requires heat [5–7]. Pyridinium salts are often formed in toluene, acetone or acetonitrile, always at high temperatures [8,9]. While designing the synthesis of a second family of derivatives acting as disease-modifying agents in Parkinson's disease [10–12], we planned as a first step the α-benzylation of commercially available methyl 2-pyridilacetate with benzyl bromide, in basic conditions, giving compound **I** (Figure 1).

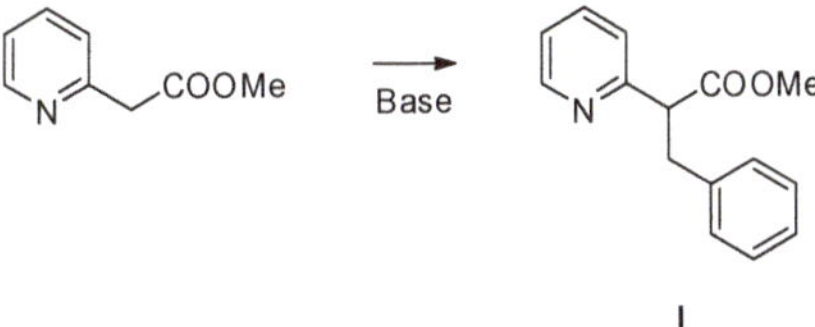

Figure 1. α-benzylation of methyl 2-pyridylacetate, the central reaction of the present work.

The main criticisms of this reaction, which affects both the overall yield and product purification, are twofold: the potential double alkylation of the α-carbon, yielding the undesired di-benzylated by-product **II**, and the benzylation of the pyridine nitrogen, with the resulting formation of the quaternary pyridinium salt **III**. The latter is particularly likely if the reaction is conducted at high temperatures. Moreover, another possibility is the initial obtainment of the desired compound **I**, followed by *N*-alkylation with unreacted benzyl bromide present in the reaction mixture, giving the by-product **IV** (Figure 2). Our

Citation: Suigo, L.; Straniero, V.; Valoti, E. 2-(1-Methoxycarbonyl-2-phenyleth-1-yl)-1-benzylpyridin-1-ium Bromide. *Molbank* **2023**, *2023*, M1738. https://doi.org/10.3390/M1738

Academic Editors: Fawaz Aldabbagh, Stefano D'Errico and Annalisa Guaragna

Received: 30 August 2023
Revised: 21 September 2023
Accepted: 12 October 2023
Published: 16 October 2023

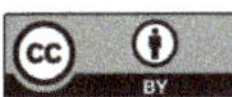

goals were to find acceptable conditions to achieve **I** with the highest possible yields while avoiding as much as possible the formation of any potential impurity, like **II**, **III** and/or **IV**.

COOMe COOMe COOMe

II **III** **IV**

Figure 2. Structures of by-products **II–IV**.

While looking for the best conditions to obtain **I**, avoiding as much as possible the formation of any by-product, we noticed how the reaction's crude product, containing only **I** and unreacted benzyl bromide, spontaneously evolved to the quantitative formation of **IV**, in a complete solvent-free environment and at room temperature, upon standing.

2. Results

To obtain compound **I**, we decided to perform the reaction between methyl 2-pyridil acetate and benzyl bromide using diisopropylethyl amine (DIPEA) as a base instead of K_2CO_3, alcoholates, LDA or sodium hexamethyldisilazane, which are more commonly used as α-alkylate esters. This choice forced us to conduct the reaction at high temperatures, due to the lower basicity of DIPEA compared to the other bases, to observe reactivity. In this regard, we found that 90 °C was the temperature at which complete consumption of methyl 2-pyridilacetate could be observed in around 7 h, although we used a double amount of benzyl bromide. In these conditions, as is typical of pyridinium salt syntheses, we expected the formation of **III** and/or **IV** as by-products. Surprisingly, no traces of **III** or **IV** were found in the ^{1}H-NMR spectrum of the crude product (Figure 3), in which only **I** and an almost equimolar amount of unreacted excess of benzyl bromide were present.

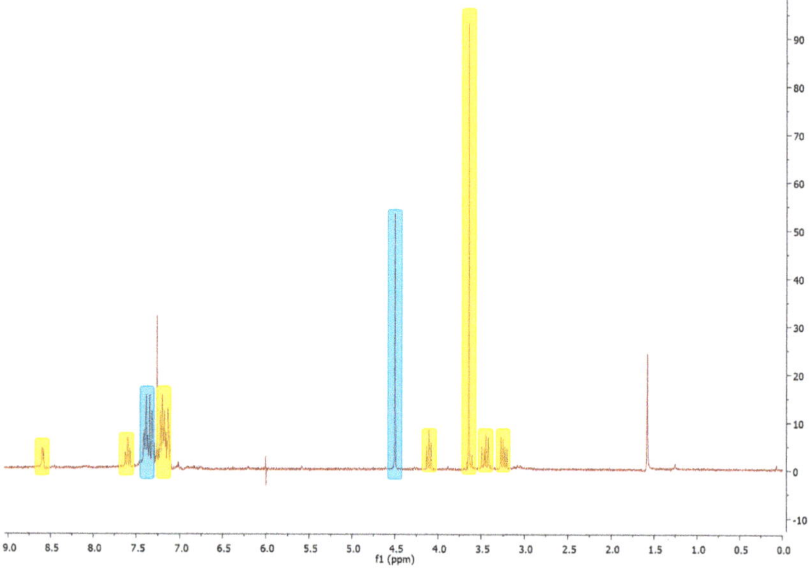

Figure 3. NMR spectrum of the crude product. NMR signals of compound **I** are highlighted in yellow, while unreacted benzyl bromide signals are marked in blue.

Thus, we decided to maintain and use these conditions to perform the reaction and, in particular, to continue along the synthetic pathway without further purification or removal of the unreacted benzyl bromide, since the following reaction should not be influenced by its presence.

Unfortunately, after 72 h, we noticed that the crude product's appearance changed from an oil to a wax and thus decided to re-check the crude product's quality via NMR. Surprisingly, we noticed how, simply upon standing at room temperature, the crude product **I** completely evolved to the formation of **IV**, which was caused by the *N*-alkylation of **I** with unreacted benzyl bromide (Figure 4).

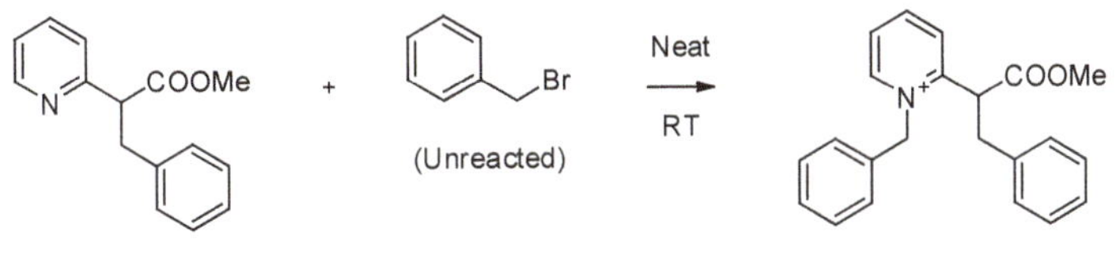

Figure 4. Conversion of **I** to **IV** in neat conditions at room temperature (RT).

The nature of the formed by-product could be easily identified by observing the number of aromatic hydrogens, the peculiar doublets of the benzyl CH_2 signal, at 6.40 and 6.17 ppm, and a shift of pyridine aromatic hydrogen signals to a higher ppm due to the EWG nature of the charged nitrogen was observed (Figure S2).

Interestingly, this quantitative conversion happened in a completely solvent-free environment and at room temperature, in reaction conditions that significantly differ from the "standard" ones employed to obtain quaternary ammonium and pyridinium salts. Then, we further confirmed compound **IV**'s nature using High-Resolution Mass Spectrometry (HRMS) analysis, which identified the expected exact mass as well as the elemental composition (Figure S4), and ^{13}C-NMR (Figure S3).

3. Material and Methods

All the reagents and solvents were acquired from commercial suppliers (Merck, Darmstadt, DE, Fluorochem, Hadfield, UK, and TCI Europe N.V., Zwijndrecht, BE) and used without further purifications. Silica gel matrix, with a fluorescent indicator of 254 nm, was used in analytical thin-layer chromatography (TLC on aluminum foils), and silica gel (particle size 40–63 μm, Merck) was used in flash chromatography with a Puriflash XS 420 (Sepachrom, Rho (Milan), Italy). Visualizations were accomplished with UV light (λ 254 or 280 nm).

The ^{1}H-NMR spectra were measured with a Varian Mercury 300 NMR spectrometer/Oxford Narrow Bore superconducting magnet operating at 300 MHz. The ^{13}C-NMR spectra were acquired at 75 MHz. Chemical shifts (δ) are reported in ppm relative to residual solvent as an internal standard. Signal multiplicity is described according to the following abbreviations: s = singlet, d = doublet, dd = doublet of doublets, ddd = doublet of doublets of doublets, dt = doublet of triplets, t = triplet and m = multiplet.

HRMS spectra were acquired with a Q-tof SYNAPT G2-Si HDMS 8K (Waters) coupled with an electrospray ionization (ESI) source in positive (ES+) ion mode.

Methyl 3-phenyl-2-(pyridin-2-yl)propanoate (I): DIPEA (1.38 mL, 7.94 mmol) and benzyl bromide (1.57 mL, 13.24 mmol) were added to a solution of methyl 2-pyridilacetate (0.89 mL, 6.62 mmol) in toluene (10 mL). The reaction mixture was heated at 90 °C and stirred for 7 h. Then, the reaction was diluted with ethyl acetate (10 mL), washed once with 10 % aqueous NaCl (20 mL), dried over Na_2SO_4, filtered and concentrated under vacuum to give 1.40 g of an orange oil corresponding to a mixture of **I** and an almost equimolar amount of unreacted benzyl bromide. ^{1}H-NMR ($CDCl_3$): δ 8.59 (ddd, J = 4.9, 1.8, 0.9 Hz,

1H), 7.61 (dt, J = 7.7, 1.8 Hz, 1H), 7.25–7.08 (m, 7H), 4.12 (t, J = 7.8 Hz, 1H), 3.64 (s, 3H), 3.46 (dd, J = 13.8, 8.0 Hz, 1H), 3.24 (dd, J = 13.8, 7.8 Hz, 1H) ppm.

2-(1-methoxycarbonyl-2-phenyleth-1-yl)-1-benzylpyridin-1-ium bromide (IV): 1.40 g of compound **IV** was obtained from the crude derivative **I**, obtained as mentioned above, upon standing in neat conditions as a yellowish oil. ^{1}H-NMR ($CDCl_3$): δ 10.20 (dd, J = 6.2, 1.1 Hz, 1H), 8.54 (dt, J = 7.9, 1.4 Hz, 1H), 8.19–8.09 (m, 2H), 7.42–7.34 (m, 3H), 7.20 (m, 3H), 7.15–7.09 (m, 2H), 6.85–6.78 (m, 2H), 6.40 (d, J = 15.6 Hz, 1H), 6.17 (d, J = 15.6 Hz, 1H), 4.60 (dd, J = 8.1, 6.9 Hz, 1H), 3.58 (s, 3H), 3.49–3.39 (m, 1H), 3.09 (dd, J = 13.7, 6.7 Hz, 1H) ppm. ^{13}C-NMR ($CDCl_3$): 168.8, 153.9, 148.5, 146.5, 135.4, 132.3, 129.7, 129.4, 129.1, 128.9, 128.8, 128.7, 127.6, 127.5, 127.2 ppm. HRMS (TOF ES+, Na+-adduct): m/z 332.1650, 333.1682. Calculated mass 332.1645, evaluated mass 332.1650.

4. Conclusions

Within this work, we report the complete and unexpected conversion of a pyridine nitrogen to a quaternary pyridinium salt at room temperature and in neat conditions without stirring. These interesting results could be further exploited for the obtainment of this important class of compounds, avoiding elevated-temperature conditions that could promote product degradation phenomena.

Supplementary Materials: The following are available online: Figure S1: ^{1}H-NMR spectrum of I. Figure S2: ^{1}H-NMR spectrum of **IV**. Figure S3: ^{13}C-NMR spectrum of **IV**. Figure S4: HRMS and elemental composition report of **IV**.

Author Contributions: L.S.: investigation, data curation, writing—original draft preparation, V.S.: supervision, project administration, writing—review and editing, resources. E.V.: conceptualization, supervision, project administration, funding acquisition. All authors have read and agreed to the published version of the manuscript.

Funding: This research received no external funding.

Data Availability Statement: Data will be made available on request.

Acknowledgments: Mass spectrometry analysis was performed at the mass spectrometry facility of Unitech COSPECT at University of Milan. The authors acknowledge the support of the APC central fund of the University of Milan.

Conflicts of Interest: The authors declare no conflict of interest.

References

1. Zhang, C.; Cui, F.; Zeng, G.; Jiang, M.; Yang, Z.; Yu, Z.; Zhu, M.; Shen, L. Quaternary ammonium compounds (QACs): A review on occurrence, fate and toxicity in the environment. *Sci. Total Environ.* **2015**, *518–519*, 352–362. [CrossRef] [PubMed]
2. Zhou, Z.; Zhou, S.; Zhang, X.; Zeng, S.; Xu, Y.; Nie, W.; Zhou, Y.; Xu, T.; Chen, P. Quaternary Ammonium Salts: Insights into Synthesis and New Directions in Antibacterial Applications. *Bioconjug. Chem.* **2023**, *34*, 302–325. [CrossRef] [PubMed]
3. Zhang, T.; Wang, K.; Ke, Y.; Tang, Y.; Liu, L.; Huang, T.; Li, C.; Tang, Z.; Chen, T. Transition-metal-free and base promoted C-C bond formation via C-N bond cleavage of organoammonium salts. *Org. Biomol. Chem.* **2021**, *19*, 8237–8240. [CrossRef] [PubMed]
4. Yang, B.; Xue, W.; Yu, B.; Pang, H.; Yu, L.; Wang, Q.; Zhu, D. Development of a Trimethylamine-Catalyzed Novel Synthesis of Azoxystrobin. *Org. Process Res. Dev.* **2023**, *27*, 1276–1282. [CrossRef]
5. Szymaniak, D.; Maćkowiak, A.; Ciarka, K.; Praczyk, T.; Marcinkowska, K.; Pernak, J. Synthesis and Characterization of Double Salt Herbicidal Ionic Liquids Comprising both 4-Chloro-2-methylphenoxyacetate and trans-Cinnamate Anions. *ChemPlusChem* **2020**, *85*, 2281–2289. [CrossRef] [PubMed]
6. Nie, L.; Yao, S.; Dong, B.; Li, X.; Song, H. Synthesis, characterization and physical properties of novel cholinium-based organic magnetic ionic liquids. *J. Mol. Liq.* **2017**, *240*, 152–161. [CrossRef]
7. Sun, J.; Zhang, S.; Cheng, W.; Ren, J. Hydroxyl-functionalized ionic liquid: A novel efficient catalyst for chemical fixation of CO_2 to cyclic carbonate. *Tetrahedron Lett.* **2008**, *49*, 3588–3591. [CrossRef]
8. Manikandan, C.; Ganesan, K. Solid-Supported Synthesis of Flexible Dimeric Pyridinium Salts and Their Catalytic Activities. *Synlett* **2016**, *27*, 1527–1530. [CrossRef]
9. Qu, B.; Mangunuru, H.P.R.; Wei, X.; Fandrick, K.R.; Desrosiers, J.-N.; Sieber, J.D.; Kurouski, D.; Haddad, N.; Samankumara, L.P.; Lee, H.; et al. Synthesis of Enantioenriched 2-Alkyl Piperidine Derivatives through Asymmetric Reduction of Pyridinium Salts. *Org. Lett.* **2016**, *18*, 4920–4923. [CrossRef] [PubMed]

10. Faustini, G.; Longhena, F.; Bruno, A.; Bono, F.; Grigoletto, J.; La Via, L.; Barbon, A.; Casiraghi, A.; Straniero, V.; Valoti, E.; et al. Alpha-synuclein/synapsin III pathological interplay boosts the motor response to methylphenidate. *Neurobiol. Dis.* **2020**, *138*, 104789. [CrossRef] [PubMed]
11. Casiraghi, A.; Longhena, F.; Faustini, G.; Ribaudo, G.; Suigo, L.; Camacho-Hernandez, G.A.; Bono, F.; Brembati, V.; Newman, A.H.; Gianoncelli, A.; et al. Methylphenidate Analogues as a New Class of Potential Disease-Modifying Agents for Parkinson's Disease: Evidence from Cell Models and Alpha-Synuclein Transgenic Mice. *Pharmaceutics* **2022**, *14*, 1595. [CrossRef] [PubMed]
12. Bellucci, A.; Casiraghi, A.; Longhena, F.; Straniero, V.; Valoti, E. Structural Analogues of Methylphenidate as Parkinson's Disease-Modifying Agents. IT202000019303A1, 5 August 2020.

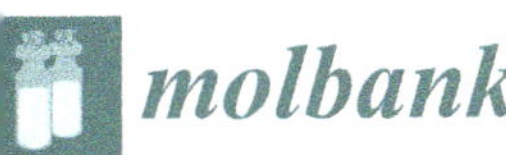 molbank

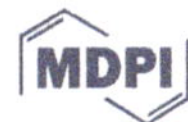

hort Note

Z)-2′-((Adamantan-1-yl)thio)-1,1′-dimethyl-2′,3′-dihydro-[2,4′-biimidazolylidene]-4,5,5′(1*H*,1′*H*,3*H*)-trione

'ladimir Burmistrov [1,2,*], Vladimir Mokhov [1], Robert R. Fayzullin [3] and Gennady M. Butov [1,2]

1 Department of Technology of Organic and Petrochemical Synthesis, Volgograd State Technical University, Volgograd 400005, Russia
2 Department of Chemistry, Technology and Equipment of Chemical Industry, Volzhsky Polytechnic Institute (Branch), Volgograd State Technical University, Volzhsky 404121, Russia
3 Arbuzov Institute of Organic and Physical Chemistry, FRC Kazan Scientific Center, Russian Academy of Sciences, 8 Arbuzov Street, Kazan 420088, Russia
* Correspondence: vburmistrov@vstu.ru

Abstract: The title compound, (*Z*)-2′-((adamantan-1-yl)thio)-1,1′-dimethyl-2′,3′-dihydro-[2,4′-biimidazolylidene]-4,5,5′(1*H*,1′*H*,3*H*)-trione, was found to be a by-product of the reaction of 1,3-dehydroadamantane with 3-methyl-2-thioxoimidazolidin-4-one and characterized via single-crystal X-ray diffraction.

Keywords: adamantane; thiohydantoin; by-product; X-ray structure

1. Introduction

2-Thioxoimidazolidin-4-one (2-thiohydantoin, Figure 1) is a very promising scaffold for the creation of biologically active compounds, with the possibility of independent functionalization in four directions [1–4]. Moreover, thiohydantoins substituted at all possible positions are available, albeit in low yields, through four-component one-pot domino-reactions [5]. However, most of the synthesized 2-thiohydantoin derivatives bear substituents in the position 3 [6,7] or 5 [8,9]. It is not surprising that many recent works have been published on the study of the biological activity of compounds derived from 2-thiohydantoin. 2-Thiohydantoin derivatives exhibit anticonvulsant [10], fungicidal [11–13], antiviral [14,15], antimutagenic [16,17], and immunomodulatory [18] bioactivities, and some of them are also considered in the hormone-independent treatment of prostate cancer [19–22].

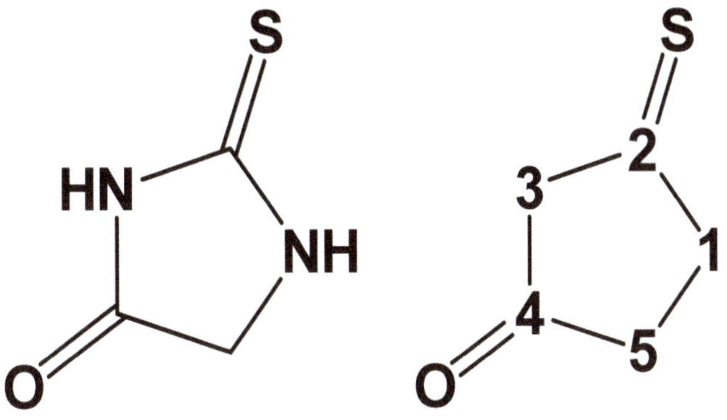

:itation: Burmistrov, V.; Mokhov, V.; ayzullin, R.R.; Butov, G.M. Z)-2′-((Adamantan-1-yl)thio)-1,1′-imethyl-2′,3′-dihydro-[2,4′-iimidazolylidene]-4,5,5′(1*H*,1′*H*,3*H*)-rione. *Molbank* **2023**, *2023*, M1585. ttps://doi.org/10.3390/M1585

cademic Editors: Stefano D'Errico nd Annalisa Guaragna

eceived: 22 January 2023
evised: 10 February 2023
ccepted: 12 February 2023
ublished: 14 February 2023

Figure 1. Structure of 2-thiohydantoin with numbered atoms.

The adamantyl fragment, due to its high lipophilicity, is part of many biologically active compounds [23]. 1,3-Dehydroadamantane (tetracyclo[$3.3.1.1^{3,7}.0^{1,3}$]decane, 1,3-

DHA, **2**, Scheme 1) is a convenient reagent for the direct introduction of the adamanty moiety into the molecules of various organic compounds with activated C–H [24] as wel as ordinary N–H bonds [25–28]. In this regard, we carried out the modification of 2 thiohydantoin and its 3-alkyl- and aryl- derivatives using 1,3-DHA. Herein, we repor a very unusual side compound obtained from the reaction of 1,3-DHA with 3-methyl-2 thioxoimidazolidin-4-one (**1**).

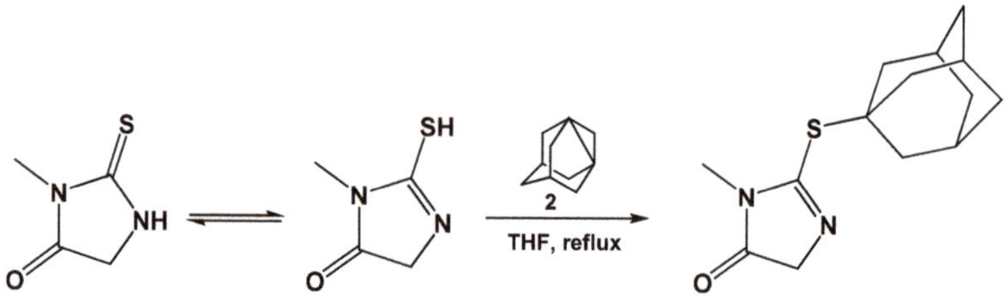

Scheme 1. Main route of the reaction of 1,3-dehydroadamantane (**2**) with 3-methyl-2-thioxoimi dazolidin-4-one (**1**).

2. Results and Discussion

It is known that 2-thiohydanoin and its 3-substituted derivatives undergo a tautomeri transformation, as is shown in Scheme 1 [29]. Thus, our study intended to establish which form of 3-methyl-2-thiohydanoin reacts with 1,3-DHA (**2**). The reaction was carried ou in THF under reflux for 8 h. We discovered that the main product of the reaction is 2 ((adamantan-1-yl)thio)-3-methyl-3,5-dihydro-4*H*-imidazol-4-one (**3**), which corresponds to the involvement of the S–H bond of **1′**, instead of the N–H of **1**.

However, during the isolation of main reaction product **3**, we found a small amoun (3%) of an unidentified by-product, which was insoluble in acetone. Separated by the filtra tion of the acetone solution, it was then dissolved in ethanol and left for slow crystallization The resulting crystals were of good quality for a single-crystal X-ray diffraction study The analysis (see supplementary) showed that the by-product was (*Z*)-2′-((adamantan 1-yl)thio)-1,1′-dimethyl-2′,3′-dihydro-[2,4′-biimidazolylidene]-4,5,5′(1*H*,1′*H*,3*H*)-trione (**5** Scheme 2, Figure 2).

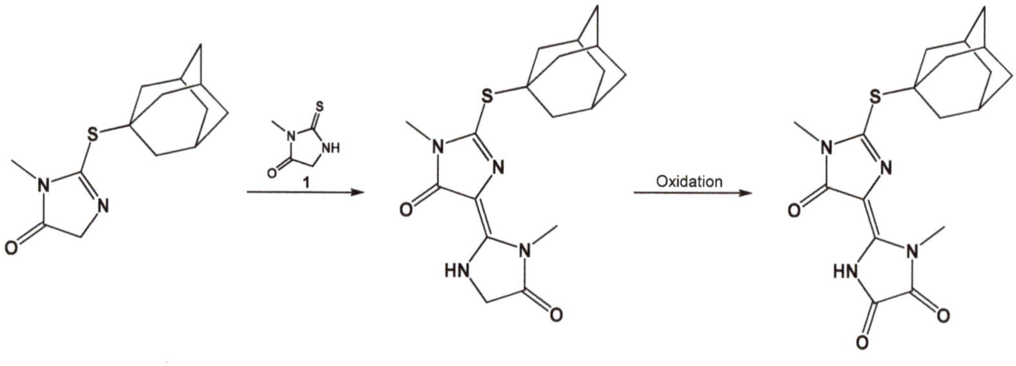

Scheme 2. Putative route of formation of the (*Z*)-2′-((adamantan-1-yl)thio)-1,1′-dimethyl-2′,3′ dihydro-[2,4′-biimidazolylidene]-4,5,5′(1*H*,1′*H*,3*H*)-trione (**5**).

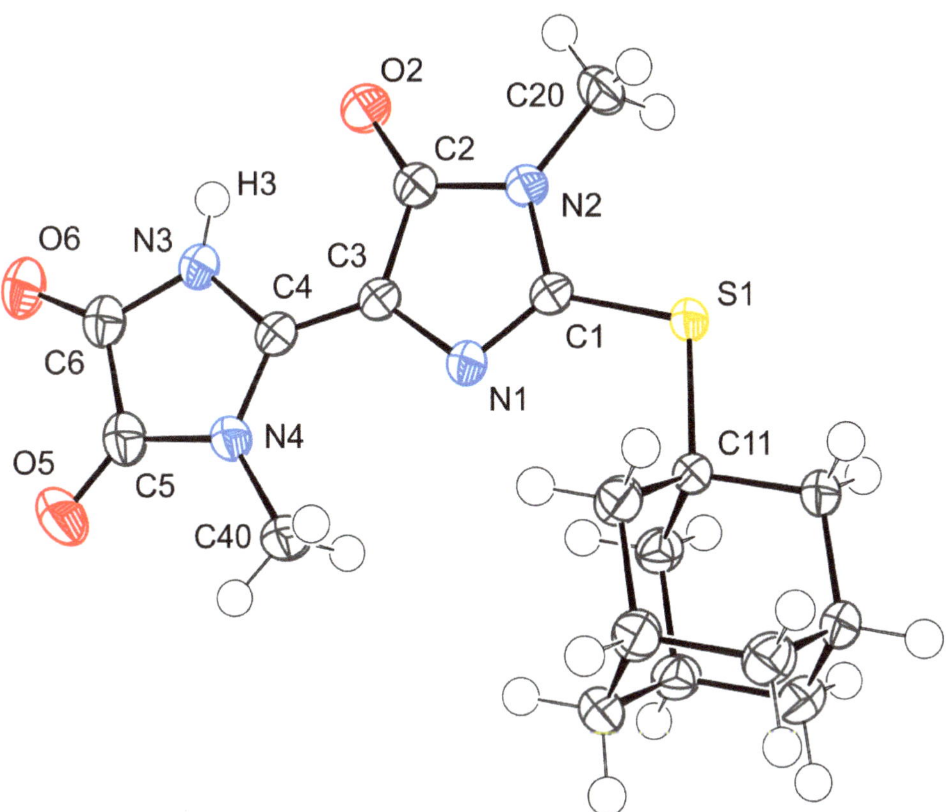

Figure 2. Structure of compound **5** in the crystal with thermal ellipsoids at the 80% probability level for nonhydrogen atoms according to single-crystal X-ray diffraction. Selected interatomic distances [Å]: S1–C1 1.7274(13), S1–C11 1.8432(13), O2–C2 1.2309(17), O5–C5 1.2087(18), O6–C6 1.2051(17), N1 C1 1.3038(17), N1 C3 1.3975(16), N2 C1 1.4032(16), N2 C2 1.3843(17), N2 C20 1.4628(17), N3 C4 1.3844(16), N3–C6 1.3734(17), N3–H3 0.86(2), N4–C4 1.3804(16), N4–C5 1.3810(17), N4–C40 1.4603(17), C2–C3 1.4660(18), C3–C4 1.3563(18), C5–C6 1.531(2).

We assume that, under the reaction conditions, main product **3** was involved in the interaction with starting compound **1** to produce a small amount of by-product **4** (Scheme 2). The reaction of 2-thiohydantoins at position 5 with carbonyl-containing compounds is well known [8,9] and the carbon atom at the position 5 of **3** could act as a potential nucleophile with respect to the thiocarbonyl group of **1**, which is present in the reaction mixture. By-product **4** could then be oxidized into **5** (Scheme 3). This fact reveals the possibility of the oligomerization of 2-thiohydanoins and should be noted in further studies as one of the yield-decreasing factors.

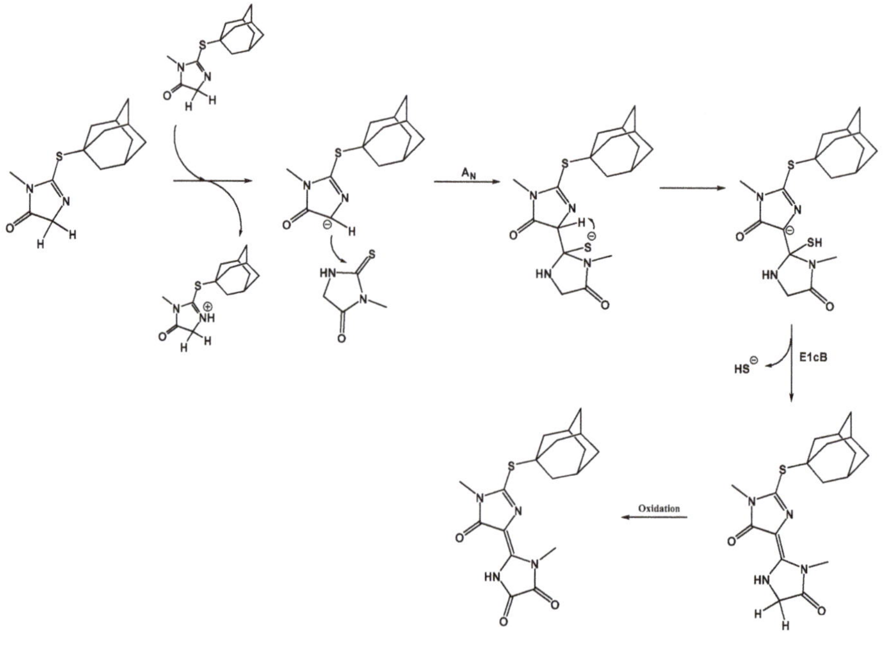

Scheme 3. Plausible mechanism for formation of compounds **4** and **5**.

3. Materials and Methods

Preparation of compound 5. A solution of 1,3-dehydroadamantane (**2**, 670 mg, 5 mmol) in 10 mL of DCM was added to the solution of 3-methyl-2-thioxoimidazolidin-4-one (**1**, 975 mg, 7.5 mmol) in 10 mL of DCM. The reaction mass was refluxed for 2 h and the solvent was removed *in vacuo*. Crude product was dissolved in acetone and filtered. Residue from the filter (35 mg) was dissolved in ethanol (2 mL) and left in a Schlenk flask for the process of slow crystallization to obtain crystals of compound **5**.

Compound **5** crystallized in the $P2_1/m$ monoclinic space group with half of the molecule in the asymmetric cell. The molecule was located on the crystallographic mirror plane. It is interesting to note that a C2–C3 bond length of 1.4660(18) Å was expected for the C(sp^2)–C(sp^2) single bond (ca. 1.47 Å), while the C5–C6 bond was noticeably longer (1.531(2) Å). The C3–C4 bond length of 1.3563(18) Å meant that it was double the expected length (ca. 1.34 Å was expected). The bond lengths of the carbonyl groups (ca. 1.21 Å was expected) were in the range from 1.2051(17) to 1.2309(17) Å. The compound was characterized by the intramolecular hydrogen bond N3–H3···O2 with the following parameters: N3–H3 0.86(2) Å, H3···O2 2.23(2) Å, N3···O2 2.8299(15) Å, and ∠N3–H3···O2 126.6(17)°. Basically, due to nonclassical hydrogen bonds C–H···O, the molecules were combined into a layer parallel to the 0*ac* plane. Then, the layers were joined together along the shortest axis 0*b* of the unit cell due to π···π interactions. The nature of nonclassical hydrogen bonds and π···π interactions in crystals was previously considered in detail [30].

The deposition number CCDC 2,234,948 contains the supplementary crystallographic data for this paper. These data are provided free of charge by the joint Cambridge Crystallographic Data Centre and Fachinformationszentrum Karlsruhe Access Structures service www.ccdc.cam.ac.uk/structures.

Single-crystal X-ray diffraction. Suitable monocrystals of **5** were prepared by slow crystallization from an ethanol solution. The data set for a single crystal **5** was collected on a Bruker D8 QUEST diffractometer with a PHOTON III area detector and an IμS

DIAMOND microfocus X-ray tube using Mo $K\alpha$ (0.71073 Å) radiation at 100(2) K. The data reduction package *APEX4* was used for data processing. Data were corrected for systematic errors and absorption: Numerical absorption correction based on integration over a multifaceted crystal model and empirical absorption correction based on spherical harmonics according to the point group symmetry $2/m$ using equivalent reflections. The structure was solved using the intrinsic phasing approach and *SHELXT*-2018/2 [31] and refined using full-matrix least-squares on F^2 using *SHELXL*-2018/3 [32]. Non-hydrogen atoms were refined anisotropically. The hydrogen atoms were found by difference Fourier maps and refined isotropically.

Crystallographic data for **5**. $C_{18}H_{22}N_4O_3S$, yellow prism (0.345 × 0.245 × 0.223 mm^3), formula weight 374.45 g mol^{-1}; monoclinic, $P2_1/m$ (No. 11), a = 11.4315(3) Å, b = 6.6765(2) Å, c = 11.5969(3) Å, β = 107.8509(5)°, V = 842.49(4) Å^3, Z = 2, Z' = 0.5, T = 100(2) K, d_{calc} = 1.476 g cm^{-3}, μ(Mo $K\alpha$) = 0.220 mm^{-1}, F(000) = 396; $T_{max/min}$ = 0.9583/0.8697; 66,553 reflections were collected (1.845° $\leq \theta \leq$ 28.304°, index ranges: $-15 \leq h \leq 15$, $-8 \leq k \leq 8$, and $-15 \leq l \leq 15$), 2268 of which were unique, R_{int} = 0.0334, R_σ = 0.0098; completeness to θ of 28.304° was 100.0%. The refinement of 198 parameters with 42 restraints converged to $R1$ = 0.0284 and $wR2$ = 0.0791 for 2195 reflections with $I > 2\sigma(I)$ and $R1$ = 0.0292 and $wR2$ = 0.0800 for all data with a goodness-of-fit of S = 1.045 and residual electron density $\rho_{max/min}$ = 0.407 and −0.215 e Å^{-3}, rms 0.045; max shift/e.s.d. in the last cycle 0.000.

4. Conclusions

In this work, we presented the previously unknown compound, (Z)-2′-((adamantan-1-yl)thio)-1,1′-dimethyl-2′,3′-dihydro-[2,4′-biimidazolylidene]-4,5,5′(1*H*,1′*H*,3*H*)-trione, which was isolated from a reaction mass and characterized by single-crystal X-ray diffraction.

Supplementary Materials: The following supporting information can be downloaded. Single-crystal X-ray diffraction data (cif).

Author Contributions: Conceptualization, V.B.; investigation, V.M. and R.R.F.; writing, review, and editing, V.B. and R.R.F.; project administration, G.M.B. All authors have read and agreed to the published version of the manuscript.

Funding: This research was performed with financial support from the Russian Science Foundation (project no. 19-73-10002). The diffraction study was carried out using equipment of the Distributed Spectral-Analytical Center of Shared Facilities for Study of Structure, Composition and Properties of Substances and Materials of FRC Kazan Scientific Center of RAS.

Data Availability Statement: Not applicable.

Conflicts of Interest: The authors declare no conflict of interest.

References

1. Wu, F.; Jiang, H.; Zheng, B.; Kogiso, M.; Yao, Y.; Zhou, C.; Li, X.; Song, Y. Inhibition of Cancer-Associated Mutant Isocitrate Dehydrogenases by 2-Thiohydantoin Compounds. *J. Med. Chem.* **2015**, *58*, 6899–6908. [CrossRef] [PubMed]
2. Gosling, S.; Rollin, P.; Tatibouët, A. Thiohydantoins: Selective N- and S-Functionalization for Liebeskind–Srogl Reaction Study. *Synthesis* **2011**, *2011*, 3649–3660.
3. Jha, S.; Silversides, J.D.; Boyle, R.W.; Archibald, S.J. Hydrogen bonded dimers vs. one-dimensional chains in 2-thiooxoimidazolidin4-one (thiohydantoin) drug derivatives. *Cryst. Eng. Comm.* **2010**, *12*, 1730–1739. [CrossRef]
4. Abou El-Regal, M.K.; Abdalha, A.A.; El-Kassaby, M.A.; Ali, A.T. Synthesis of New Thiohydantoin Derivatives Under Phase Transfer Catalysis. *Phosphorus Sulfur Silicon* **2007**, *182*, 845–851. [CrossRef]
5. Renault, S.; Bertrand, S.; Carreaux, F.; Bazureau, J.P. Parallel Solution-Phase Synthesis of 2-Alkylthio-5-arylidene-3,5-dihydro-4H-imidazol-4-one by One-Pot Three-Component Domino Reaction. *J. Comb. Chem.* **2007**, *9*, 935–942. [CrossRef]
6. Burmistrov, V.V.; Pitushkin, D.A.; Vasipov, V.V.; D'yachenko, V.S.; Butov, G.M. Synthesis of 3-adamantylated hydantoins and their 2-thio(seleno) analogs. *Chem. Heterocycl. Comp.* **2019**, *55*, 619–622. [CrossRef]
7. Burmistrov, V.; Saxena, R.; Pitushkin, D.; Butov, G.M.; Chung, F.-L.; Aggarwal, M. Adamantyl Isothiocyanates as Mutant p53 Rescuing Agents and Their Structure−Activity Relationships. *J. Med. Chem.* **2021**, *64*, 6621–6633. [CrossRef]

8. Beloglazkina, E.K.; Majouga, A.G.; Yudin, I.V.; Frolova, N.A.; Zyk, N.V.; Dolzhikova, V.D.; Moiseeva, A.A.; Rakhimov, R.D.; Butin, K.P. 5-(Pyridylmethylidene)-substituted 2-thiohydantoins and their complexes with Cu^{II}, Ni^{II}, and Co^{II}: Synthesis, electrochemical study, and adsorption on the cystamine-modified gold surface. *Russ. Chem. Bull.* **2006**, *55*, 1015–1027. [CrossRef]
9. Sirivolu, V.R.; Vernekar, S.K.V.; Marchand, C.; Naumova, A.; Chergui, A.; Renaud, A.; Stephen, A.G.; Chen, F.; Sham, Y.Y.; Pommier, Y.; et al. 5-Arylidenethioxothiazolidinones as Inhibitors of Tyrosyl–DNA Phosphodiesterase I. *J. Med. Chem.* **2012**, *55*, 8671–8684. [CrossRef]
10. Dang, P.; Madan, A.K. Structure-Activity Study on Anticonvulsant (Thio) Hydantoins Using Molecular Connectivity Indices. *J. Chem. Inf. Comput. Sci.* **1994**, *34*, 1162–1166. [CrossRef]
11. Lindel, T.; Hoffmann, H. Synthesis of dispacamide from the marine sponge *agelas dispar*. *Tetrahedron Lett.* **1997**, *38*, 8935–8938. [CrossRef]
12. Yadav, L.D.S.; Shukla, S. Synthesis of new peptidyl imidazodithi(and -thiadi)azoles as potential fungicides. *J. Agric. Food Chem.* **1995**, *43*, 2526–2529. [CrossRef]
13. Marton, J.; Enisz, J.; Hosztafi, S.; Timar, T. Preparation and fungicidal activity of 5-substituted hydantoins and their 2-thio analogs. *J. Agric. Food Chem.* **1993**, *41*, 148–152. [CrossRef]
14. Yong, X.; Su, M.; Wan, W.; You, W.; Lu, X.; Qu, J.; Liu, R. 2-Thiohydantoin containing OH and NH recognition subunits: A fluoride ion selective colorimetric sensor. *New J. Chem.* **2013**, *37*, 1591–1594. [CrossRef]
15. El-Barbary, A.A.; Khodair, A.I.; Pedersen, E.B.; Nielsen, C. S-Glucosylated hydantoins as new antiviral agents. *J. Med. Chem.* **1994**, *37*, 73–77. [CrossRef]
16. Takahashi, A.; Matsuoka, H.; Ozawa, Y.; Uda, Y. Antimutagenic Properties of 3,5-Disubstituted 2-Thiohydantoins. *J. Agric. Food Chem.* **1998**, *46*, 5037–5042. [CrossRef]
17. Froelich, E.; Fruehan, A.; Jackman, M.; Kirchner, F.K.; Alexander, E.J.; Archer, S. 5-Heptyl-2-Thiohydantoin, a New Antitubercular Agent. *J. Am. Chem. Soc.* **1954**, *76*, 3099–3100. [CrossRef]
18. Blanc, M.; Cussac, M.; Boucherle, A.; Leclerc, G. Synthesis and immunomodulating activity of 1-amino-2-thiohydantoin derivatives. *Eur. J. Med. Chem.* **1992**, *27*, 839–843. [CrossRef]
19. Tran, C.; Ouk, S.; Clegg, N.J.; Chen, Y.; Watson, P.A.; Arora, V.; Wongvipat, J.; Smith-Jones, P.M.; Yoo, D.; Kwon, A.; et al. Development of a Second-Generation Antiandrogen for Treatment of Advanced Prostate Cancer. *Science* **2009**, *324*, 787–790. [CrossRef]
20. Taplin, M.-E.; Balk, S.P. Androgen receptor: A key molecule in the progression of prostate cancer to hormone independence. *J. Cell. Biochem.* **2004**, *91*, 483–490. [CrossRef]
21. Harrison, C. New approaches to anti-androgen activities. *Nat. Rev. Drug Discov.* **2009**, *8*, 452–453. [CrossRef]
22. Shen, H.C.; Balk, S.P. Development of androgen receptor antagonists with promising activity in castration-resistant prostate cancer. *Cancer Cell* **2009**, *15*, 461–463. [CrossRef]
23. Wanka, L.; Iqbal, K.; Schreiner, P.R. The Lipophilic Bullet Hits the Targets: Medicinal Chemistry of Adamantane Derivatives. *Chem. Rev.* **2013**, *113*, 3516–3604. [CrossRef] [PubMed]
24. Mokhov, V.M.; Butov, G.M. Adamantylation of Carbonitriles with 1,3-Dehydroadamantane and Its Homologs. *Russ. J. Org. Chem.* **2014**, *50*, 1279–1282. [CrossRef]
25. Butov, G.M.; Mokhov, V.M.; Parshin, G.Y.; Panyushkina, O.A. Adamantylation of Azoles by 1,3-Dehydroadamantane: I. N-Adamantylation of Imidazoles by 1,3-Dehydroadamantane. *Russ. J. Org. Chem.* **2009**, *45*, 1732–1733. [CrossRef]
26. Butov, G.M.; Mokhov, V.M. Reaction of 1,3-Dehydroadamantane with Dicarboxylic Acid Imides. *Russ. J. Org. Chem.* **2013**, *49*, 1403–1404. [CrossRef]
27. No, B.I.; Mokhov, V.M.; Vishnevetskii, E.N. Preparation of Adamantyl-substituted Amino Acids Lactams. *Russ. J. Org. Chem.* **2003**, *39*, 1193–1194. [CrossRef]
28. Butov, G.M.; Mokhov, V.M.; Burmistrov, V.V.; Saad, K.R.; Pitushkin, D.A. Reactions of 1,3-dehydroadamantane with inorganic oxygen-free acids. *Russ. J. Org. Chem.* **2014**, *50*, 1276–1278. [CrossRef]
29. Dürüst, Y.; Nohut, F. A New And Convenient Synthesis Of Some Substituted Thiohydantoins. *Synth. Commun.* **1999**, *29*, 1997–2005. [CrossRef]
30. Shteingolts, S.A.; Stash, A.I.; Tsirelson, V.G.; Fayzullin, R.R. Orbital-Free Quantum Crystallographic View on Noncovalent Bonding: Insights into Hydrogen Bonds, $\pi\cdots\pi$ and Reverse Electron Lone Pair$\cdots\pi$ Interactions. *Chem. Eur. J.* **2021**, *27*, 7789–7809. [CrossRef]
31. Sheldrick, G.M. SHELXT—Integrated Space-Group and Crystal-Structure Determination. *Acta Crystallogr. Sect. A Found. Adv.* **2015**, *71*, 3–8. [CrossRef] [PubMed]
32. Sheldrick, G.M. Crystal Structure Refinement with SHELXL. *Acta Crystallogr. Sect. C Struct. Chem.* **2015**, *71*, 3–8. [CrossRef] [PubMed]

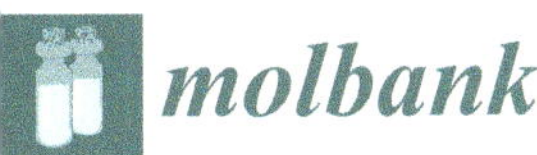 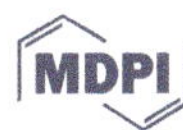

Communication

Manganese(II) Bromide Coordination toward the Target Product and By-Product of the Condensation Reaction between 2-Picolylamine and Acenaphthenequinone

Vera V. Khrizanforova, Robert R. Fayzullin and Yulia H. Budnikova *

Arbuzov Institute of Organic and Physical Chemistry, FRC Kazan Scientific Center, Russian Academy of Sciences, 8 Arbuzov Street, Kazan 420088, Russia; khrizanforovavera@yandex.ru (V.V.K.); robert.fayzullin@gmail.com (R.R.F.)
* Correspondence: yulia@iopc.ru

Abstract: A heteroleptic binuclear manganese complex was obtained and characterized by single-crystal X-ray diffraction. Manganese ions coordinate with the target product and by-product of the condensation reaction between 2-picolylamine and acenaphthenequinone are characterized by different geometries in the resulting complex.

Keywords: alkyl-BIAN; picolylamine; manganese; condensation reaction; acenaphthenequinone; X-ray structure

Citation: Khrizanforova, V.V.; Fayzullin, R.R.; Budnikova, Y.H. Manganese(II) Bromide Coordination toward the Target Product and By-Product of the Condensation Reaction between 2-Picolylamine and Acenaphthenequinone. *Molbank* **2023**, *2023*, M1606. https://doi.org/10.3390/M1606

Academic Editors: Stefano D'Errico and Annalisa Guaragna

Received: 27 February 2023
Revised: 20 March 2023
Accepted: 20 March 2023
Published: 22 March 2023

1. Introduction

Transition metal complexes with bis-iminoacenaphthenes (BIANs) are found in application in different areas of modern chemistry [1]; for instance, they serve as catalysts for many types of organic reactions [2–6] and act as magnetoactive [7,8] and optical [9] materials. Manganese complexes are of special interest because of their potential activity in small molecule activation [10].

The synthesis of alkyl-BIANs is often complicated by side reactions occurring between alkyl-substituted primary amines and acenaphthenequinone (AQ) [11–16]. This is the reason for a limited number of known, well-characterized alkyl-BIANs. Sometimes, the reaction of primary alkyl amine with AQ leads to a large number of by-products, whereas the desired product is practically absent. For example, as a result of the reaction of AQ with benzylamine, the authors identified several by-products, as shown in Scheme 1 [11–16]. This behavior can be explained by a set of isomerization/tautomerization, oxidation, and hydrolysis reactions during the treatment of primary aliphatic amine and AQ.

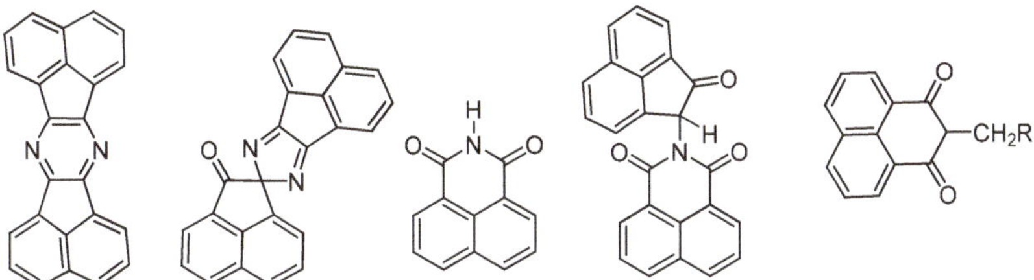

Scheme 1. Possible by-products of the reaction between aliphatic amine and AQ according to the literature.

2. Results

In this work, we performed an *in situ* condensation reaction between 2-picolylamine and AQ. Our efforts to purify the reaction mixture by column chromatography failed because of air sensitivity and the formation of an insoluble resinous precipitate. Therefore, we carried out an *in situ* chemical reduction of the crude reaction mixture obtained in the previous step by metallic sodium (1.1 equiv. per 1 mol of initial AQ) in an inert nitrogen atmosphere. After sodium was fully dissolved, manganese(II) bromide was added. The resulting product was crystallized to give manganese complex **1**. Isolated complex **1** demonstrated EPR silence at room temperature. The ^{1}H NMR spectrum of complex **1** was also not informative because of the broadening of proton signals (see Supplementary Materials). We managed to describe the molecular structure of **1** by single-crystal X-ray diffraction. Thus, it was found that neutral binuclear complex **1** contained not only the target mono-iminoacenaphthene ligand (L_1) but also an unexpected 14-(pyridin-2-yl)-14*H*-acenaphtho[1,2-*b*]naphtho[1,8-*fg*]quinoxalin-14-ol ligand (L_2). The overall reaction scheme and structural formula of the final product are shown in Scheme 2.

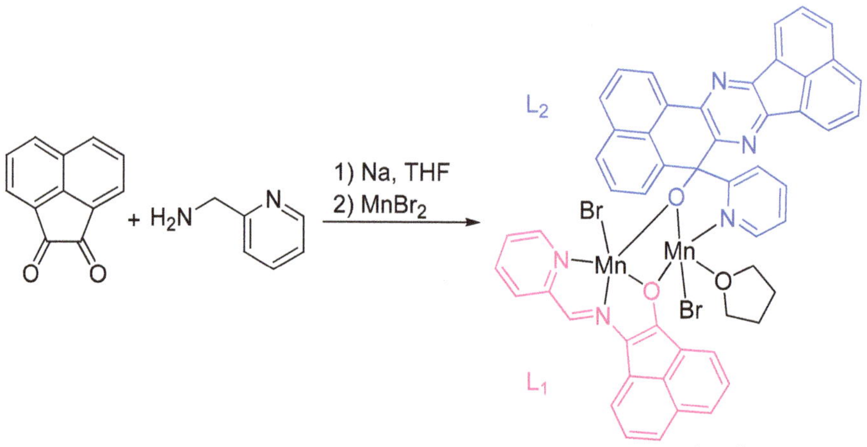

Scheme 2. Synthesis of binuclear manganese complex **1**.

Complex **1** crystallized in the triclinic space group $P\bar{1}$ with tetrahydrofuran (THF) solvent molecules. According to X-ray diffraction data, compound **1** was a neutral binuclear complex with the Mn1···Mn2 internuclear distance of 3.2818(7) Å, indicating the absence of metal–metal bonding, as shown in Figure 1. The manganese atoms differed in their coordination geometry, namely, the atom Mn1 adopted distorted square pyramidal coordination with geometry index [17] τ_5 = 0.19, while the atom Mn2 was close to octahedral one if the elongated coordination bond Mn2–N3 of 2.493(3) Å was taken into account. The ligand L_1 was coordinated by Mn1 via the atoms O1, N1, and N2, whereas the ligand L_2 bound Mn2 through the atoms N3, N5, and O2 as well as Mn1 through the oxygen atom O2. Internuclear distances of the coordination sphere are listed in the figure caption. The positions of the hydrogen atoms of **1** were confirmed by Fourier maps and corresponded to the skeletal formula in Scheme 2. The analysis of bond lengths within the ligand L_1 in complex **1** showed the migration of double bond from N1–C102 (1.369(5) Å) to N1–C21 (1.289(5) Å). The charge distribution analysis showed that L_2 was an anion with a formal negative charge of −1 on oxygen atom O2. The ligand L_1 also demonstrated anionic character.

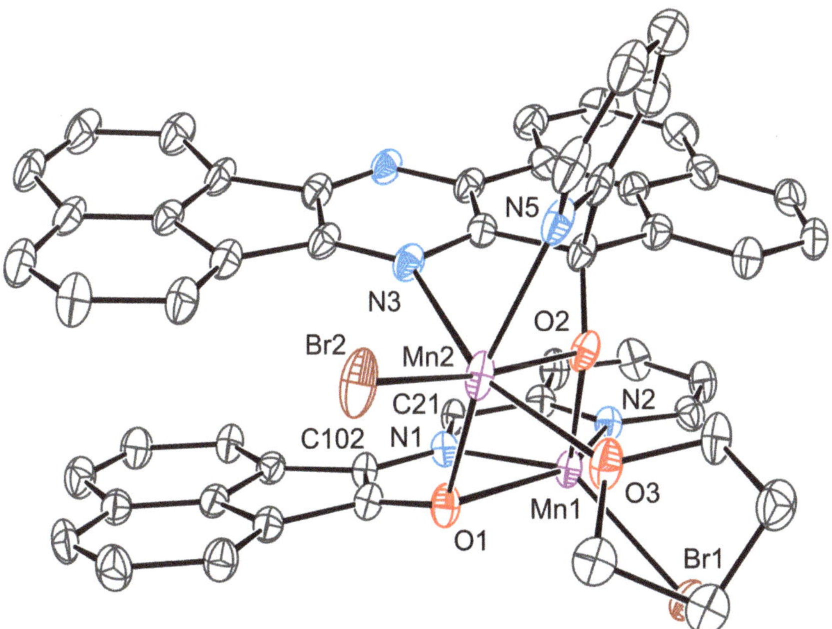

Figure 1. Molecular structure of **1** in the crystal with thermal ellipsoids at the 50% probability level according to single-crystal X-ray diffraction. Hydrogen atoms and solvent molecules are omitted for clarity. Selected interatomic distances [Å]: Br1–Mn1 2.4871(7), Mn1–O1 2.316(3), Mn1–O2 2.031(3), Mn1–N1 2.191(3), Mn1–N2 2.265(3), Br2–Mn2 2.5335(7), Mn2–O1 2.208(3), Mn2–O2 2.139(3), Mn2–O3 2.199(3), Mn2–N3 2.493(3), Mn2–N5 2.264(4).

3. Materials and Methods

Preparation. All manipulations were carried out under nitrogen, using the standard Schlenk technique or in a glove box. The solvents (THF and hexane) were distilled from sodium/benzophenone and stored over 3 Å molecular sieves under nitrogen gas. Acenaphthenequinone (95%, CAS—82-86-0), 2-aminomethyl-pyridine (99%, CAS 3731-51-9), and manganese(II) bromide $MnBr_2$ (98%, CAS 13446-03-2) were purchased and used without preliminary purification.

Synthesis of manganese complex **1**. A solution of 1 equivalent of 2-aminomethyl-pyridine (5 mmol, 0.54 g) in 3 mL of THF was dropwise added to a solution of 1 equivalent of acenaphthenequinone (5 mmol, 0.91 g) in 30 mL of THF. The reaction mixture was stirred at room temperature for about 24 h. Then, metallic sodium (1.1 equiv., 0.0023 g) was added and the solution was stirred for another 24 h. After that, manganese(II) bromide was added in one portion to the reaction mixture and, after 3 h of intense stirring, the solution was filtered. The filtrate was concentrated under a vacuum.

Single-crystal X-ray diffraction. The monocrystal analyzed was obtained by slow diffusion of *n*-hexane in THF at −35 °C. The diffraction data of **1** were registered on a Bruker D8 QUEST diffractometer with a PHOTON III area detector and an IμS DIAMOND microfocus X-ray tube using Mo $K\alpha$ (0.71073 Å) radiation at 105(2) K. The data reduction package *APEX*4 was used for data processing. The data collected were corrected for systematic errors and absorption: empirical absorption correction based on spherical harmonics according to the Laue symmetry $\overline{1}$ using equivalent reflections. The structure was solved by the direct methods using *SHELXT*-2018/2 [18] and refined by the full-matrix least-squares on F^2 using *SHELXL*-2018/3 [19]. Non-hydrogen atoms were refined anisotropically. The hydrogen atoms were found by Fourier maps, inserted at the calculate positions, and refined as riding atoms.

Crystallographic data for **1**. $C_{58}H_{47}Br_2Mn_2N_5O_{4.5}$, plate (0.098 × 0.012 × 0.007 mm^3), formula weight 1155.70 g mol^{-1}; triclinic, $P\bar{1}$ (No. 2), a = 11.4754(3) Å, b = 13.0017(4) Å, c = 16.9515(5) Å, α = 90.9576(10)°, β = 103.9529(10)°, γ = 90.4510(11)°, V = 2454.01(12) $Å^3$, Z = 2, Z' = 1, T = 105(2) K, d_{calc} = 1.564 g cm^{-3}, μ(Mo $K\alpha$) = 2.199 mm^{-1}, $F(000)$ = 1172, $T_{max/min}$ = 0.9281/0.8469; 64665 reflections were collected (1.945° ≤ θ ≤ 25.349°, inde ranges: $-13 \leq h \leq 13$, $-15 \leq k \leq 15$, and $-20 \leq l \leq 20$), 8993 of which were unique R_{int} = 0.0749, R_σ = 0.0455; completeness to θ of 25.349° 100.0%. The refinement of 713 parameters with 324 restraints converged to $R1$ = 0.0430 and $wR2$ = 0.1065 for 6802 reflections with $I > 2\sigma(I)$ and $R1$ = 0.0636 and $wR2$ = 0.1180 for all data with goodness-of-fit S = 1.05 and residual electron density $\rho_{max/min}$ = 1.091 and −0.565 e $Å^{-3}$, rms 0.091; max shift/e.s.d in the last cycle 0.001.

Deposition number CCDC 2244472 contains the supplementary crystallographic data for this paper. These data are provided free of charge by the joint Cambridge Crystallographic Data Centre and Fachinformationszentrum Karlsruhe Access Structures service www.ccdc.cam.ac.uk/structures (accessed on 24 February 2023).

4. Conclusions

Thus, a new binuclear manganese complex with two different N,O-ligands was obtained and structurally characterized by single-crystal X-ray diffraction. An interesting ligand environment near two manganese centers possibly makes this complex promising for further application in small molecule activation reactions.

Supplementary Materials: The following supporting information can be downloaded: EPR spectrum, ^{1}H NMR spectrum, and crystallographic data in Crystallographic Information File (CIF) format.

Author Contributions: V.V.K., conceptualization, investigation, writing—original draft preparation; R.R.F., conceptualization, formal analysis, investigation, writing—original draft preparation, visualization, data curation; Y.H.B., writing—review and editing, supervision. All authors discussed and approved the final version. All authors have read and agreed to the published version of the manuscript.

Funding: The work was supported by the Russian Science Foundation (Grant No. 21-73-10186). The authors gratefully acknowledge the Assigned Spectral Analytical Center of FRC Kazan Scientific Center of RAS for providing the necessary facilities to carry out physical-chemical measurements.

Data Availability Statement: Data are contained within the article and the Supplementary Materials.

Conflicts of Interest: The authors declare no conflict of interest.

References

1. Gasperini, M.; Ragaini, F.; Cenini, S. Synthesis of Ar-BIAN Ligands (Ar-BIAN = Bis(aryl)acenaphthenequinonediimine) Having Strong Electron-Withdrawing Substituents on the Aryl Rings and Their Relative Coordination Strength toward Palladium(0) and -(II) Complexes. *Organometallics* **2002**, *21*, 2950–2957. [CrossRef]
2. Fedushkin, I.L.; Kazarina, O.V.; Lukoyanov, A.N.; Skatova, A.A.; Bazyakina, N.L.; Cherkasov, A.V.; Palamidis, E. Mononuclear dpp-Bian Gallium Complexes: Synthesis, Crystal Structures, and Reactivity toward Alkynes and Enones. *Organometallics* **2015**, *34*, 1498–1506. [CrossRef]
3. Gottumukkala, A.L.; Teichert, J.F.; Heijnen, D.; Eisink, N.; Dijk, S.; Ferrer, C.; Hoogenband, A.; Minnaard, A.J. Pd-Diimine: A Highly Selective Catalyst System for the Base-Free Oxidative Heck Reaction. *J. Org. Chem.* **2011**, *76*, 3498–3501. [CrossRef] [PubMed]
4. Villa, M.; Miesel, D.; Hildebrandt, A.; Ragaini, F.; Schaarschmidt, D.; Wangelin, A.J. Synthesis and Catalysis of Redox-Active Bis(imino)acenaphthene (BIAN) Iron Complexes. *ChemCatChem* **2017**, *9*, 3203–3209. [CrossRef]
5. Hazari, A.S.; Ray, R.; Hoque, M.A.; Lahiri, G.K. Electronic Structure and Multicatalytic Features of Redox-Active Bis(arylimino)acenaphthene (BIAN)-Derived Ruthenium Complexes. *Inorg. Chem.* **2016**, *55*, 8160–8173. [CrossRef] [PubMed]
6. Soshnikov, I.E.; Bryliakov, K.P.; Antonov, A.A.; Sun, W.-H.; Talsi, E.P. Ethylene Polymerization of Nickel Catalysts with α-Diimine Ligands: Factors Controlling the Structure of Active Species and Polymer Properties. *Dalton Trans.* **2019**, *48*, 7974–7984. [CrossRef] [PubMed]

7. Yambulatov, D.S.; Nikolaevskii, S.A.; Kiskin, M.A.; Magdesieva, T.V.; Levitskiy, O.A.; Korchagin, D.V.; Efimov, N.N.; Vasil'ev, P.N.; Goloveshkin, A.S.; Sidorov, A.A.; et al. Complexes of Cobalt(II) Iodide with Pyridine and Redox Active 1,2-Bis(arylimino)acenaphthene: Synthesis, Structure, Electrochemical, and Single Ion Magnet Properties. *Molecules* **2020**, *25*, 2054. [CrossRef] [PubMed]
8. Yambulatov, D.S.; Nikolaevskii, S.A.; Kiskin, M.A.; Kholin, K.V.; Khrizanforov, M.N.; Yu, G.; Babeshkin, K.A.; Efimov, N.N.; Goloveshkin, A.S.; Imshennik, V.K.; et al. Generation of a Hetero Spin Complex from Iron(II) Iodide with Redox Active Acenaphthene-1,2-Diimine. *Molecules* **2021**, *26*, 2998. [CrossRef] [PubMed]
9. Hay, M.A.; Janetzki, J.T.; Kumar, V.J.; Gable, R.W.; Clérac, R.; Starikova, A.A.; Low, P.J.; Boskovic, C. Modulation of Charge Distribution in Cobalt-α-Diimine Complexes toward Valence Tautomerism. *Inorg. Chem.* **2022**, *61*, 17609–17622. [CrossRef] [PubMed]
10. Kaim, V.; Kaur-Ghumaan, S. Manganese Complexes: Hydrogen Generation and Oxidation. *Eur. J. Inorg. Chem.* **2019**, *2019*, 5041–5051. [CrossRef]
11. Moore, J.A.; Vasudevan, K.; Hill, N.J.; Reeske, G.; Cowley, A.H. Facile routes to Alkyl-BIAN ligands. *Chem. Commun.* **2006**, *27*, 2913–2915. [CrossRef] [PubMed]
12. Ragaini, F.; Gasperini, M.; Parma, P.; Gallo, E.; Casati, N.; Macchi, P. Stability-inducing strain: Application to the synthesis of alkyl-BIAN ligands (alkyl-BIAN = bis(alkyl)acenaphthenequinonediimine). *New J. Chem.* **2006**, *30*, 1046–1057. [CrossRef]
13. Ragaini, F.; Gasperini, M.; Gallo, E.; Macchi, P. Using ring strain to inhibit a decomposition path: First synthesis of an Alkyl-BIAN ligand (Alkyl-BIAN = bis(alkyl)acenaphthenequinonediimine). *Chem. Commun.* **2005**, 1031–1033. [CrossRef] [PubMed]
14. Hagar, M.; Ragaini, F.; Monticelli, E.; Caselli, A.; Macchi, P.; Casati, N. Chiral cyclopropylamines in the synthesis of new ligands; first asymmetric Alkyl-BIAN compounds. *Chem. Commun.* **2010**, *46*, 6153–6155. [CrossRef] [PubMed]
15. Tsuge, O.; Tashiro, M. Studies of Acenaphthene Derivatives. XI. The Reaction of Acenaphthenequinone with Aliphatic Amines. *Bull. Chem. Soc. Jpn.* **1965**, *38*, 399–402. [CrossRef]
16. Tsuge, O.; Tashiro, M. Studies of Acenaphthene Derivatives. XII. On the Red Substance Obtained from Acenaphthenequinone and Ammonia. *Bull. Chem. Soc. Jpn.* **1966**, *39*, 2477–2479. [CrossRef]
17. Addison, A.W.; Rao, T.N.; Reedijk, J.; van Rijn, J.; Verschoor, G.C. Synthesis, structure, and spectroscopic properties of copper(II) compounds containing nitrogen–sulphur donor ligands; the crystal and molecular structure of aqua[1,7-bis(N-methylbenzimidazol-2′-yl)-2,6-dithiaheptane]copper(II) perchlorate. *J. Chem. Soc. Dalton Trans.* **1984**, *7*, 1349–1356. [CrossRef]
18. Sheldrick, G.M. *SHELXT*—Integrated Space-Group and Crystal-Structure Determination. *Acta Crystallogr. Sect. A Found. Adv.* **2015**, *71*, 3–8. [CrossRef] [PubMed]
19. Sheldrick, G.M. Crystal Structure Refinement with *SHELXL*. *Acta Crystallogr. Sect. C Struct. Chem.* **2015**, *71*, 3–8. [CrossRef] [PubMed]

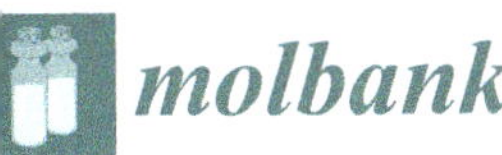 molbank 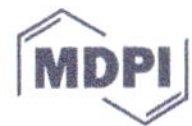

ommunication

Diethyl 2-((aryl(alkyl)amino)methylene)malonates: Unreported Mycelial Growth Inhibitors against *Fusarium oxysporum*

Villy-Fernando Cely-Veloza *, Diego Quiroga and Ericsson Coy-Barrera *

Bioorganic Chemistry Laboratory, Facultad de Ciencias Básicas y Aplicadas, Universidad Militar Nueva Granada, Cajicá 250247, Colombia

* Correspondence: u7700102@unimilitar.edu.co (W.-F.C.-V.); ericsson.coy@unimilitar.edu.co (E.C.-B.)

Abstract: This paper presents the discovery and development of antifungal agents against *Fusarium oxysporum* (*Fox*), a devastating plant pathogen. Diethyl 2-((arylamino)methylene)malonates (DAMMs) were formed as side-products during the synthesis of polysubstituted-2-pyridones through a three-component domino reaction and seemed to have antifungal activity against *Fox*. DAMMs are typically employed as intermediates or precursors to produce further bioactive compounds, but they have never been examined as antifungals. To confirm this latter characteristic, we employed a single-step procedure (i.e., the first step of the Gould-Jacobs reaction) to prepare five DAMMs (74–96% yields) which were subsequently evaluated against *Fox* in terms of their abilities to inhibit mycelial growth. The antifungal outcome was promising (0.013 µM < IC_{50} < 35 µM), involving fungistatic or fungicide effects. This small group of active compounds showed differences in antifungal activity, constituting the basis of further studies to expand the DAMM chemical space and look for improved antifungal activity.

Keywords: enamine esters; microwave; antifungals; *Fusarium oxysporum*

:itation: Cely-Veloza, W.-F.; Quiroga,).; Coy-Barrera, E. Diethyl 2-aryl(alkyl)amino)methylene)malon tes: Unreported Mycelial Growth nhibitors against *Fusarium xysporum*. *Molbank* **2023**, *2023*, 11630. https://doi.org/10.3390/11630

cademic Editor: Bartolo Gabriele

eceived: 21 February 2023
evised: 10 April 2023
ccepted: 19 April 2023
ublished: 23 April 2023

1. Introduction

Plant pathogens are a relevant problem in commercial crops, mainly related to emergence resistance; therefore, discovering and developing new antifungal agents is currently needed [1]. Among problematic phytopathogens, *Fusarium oxysporum* (*Fox*) is a case of interest as an opportunistic microorganism and devastating plant pathogen [2]. As part of our research on compounds against fungal phytopathogens, during the synthesis of polysubstituted-2-pyridones (PS2Ps) using a three-component domino reaction between diethyl ethoxymethylenemalonate (DEEMM), primary amines, and 1,3-dicarbonyl compounds (1,3-DCs) [3], diethyl 2-((ary(alkyl)lamino)methylene)malonates (DAMMs) were formed as side-products by varying the electrophilic nature of the 1,3-DC; this phenomenon was previously unreported for this domino reaction. Notably, amines first reacted with DEEMM instead of the low-electrophilic 1,3-DC (Scheme 1).

Scheme 1. Three-component domino reaction between diethyl ethoxymethylenemalonate (DEEMM), primary amines, and 1,3-dicarbonyl compounds (1,3-DCs) [3] to produce polysubstituted-2-pyridones (PS2Ps) (main product) and diethyl 2-((arylamino)methylene)malonates (DAMMs) (side-product).

Apart from the moderate scope involved in forming these side-products, they caught our attention, since partially depurated target compounds contaminated with DAMMs exhibited higher antifungal activity against *Fox* than entirely-purified PS2Ps. This fact promoted our interest in deepening the antifungal activity of DAMMs as bioactive compounds against *Fox*.

DAMMs are chemically characterized as symmetric diesters containing an aromatic substituted enamine group. They are part of a relevant group of organic compounds that have been used as intermediates or precursors for the synthesis of biologically-active compounds such as quinolones [4], β-oxocarboxylic acids [5], 2,2-*bis*(ethoxycarbonyl)vinylamine derivatives [6], 4-oxoquinoline-3-carboxamide derivatives [7], amido-esters [8], enamine esters [9], functionalized malonic acid half ester [10], 3-formyl-4(1*H*)-pyridones [11], and pyrimidinones [12].

Various protocols have been developed to synthesize DAMMs. They are primarily based on the reaction of anilines with in situ or previously generated electron-deficient olefins, comprising moderate-to-good yields (>50%). For instance, a multicomponent reaction between substituted anilines, diethyl malonate, ethyl orthoformate, acetic anhydride and catalytic amounts of $ZnCl_2$ or $FeCl_3$ was reported in the 1980s to afford DAMMs (50–85% yield) (Scheme A1a) [13,14]. The base-catalyzed trichloromethyl elimination from diethyl 2-(2,2,2-trifluoro-1-(phenylamino)ethyl)malonate, previously prepared from a two-step procedure, was also reported to produce DAMMs with good three-step overall yields (>70%) (Scheme A1b) [9]. However, the first-reported strategy to prepare DAMMs is the most widely studied procedure, based on the first step of the Gould-Jacobs reaction (reported in the 1930s) and initially performed to obtain quinolines and 4-hydroxyquinoline derivatives [15]. This Gould-Jacobs-based first step involves the thermal reaction of anilines with alkoxy methylene malonic esters or acyl malonic esters [16]. DEEMM is commercially available and is a commonly used electron-deficient olefin. It was used for this reaction with anilines and other nucleophiles since it is a versatile Michael addition acceptor [17]. This thermal addition-elimination over DEEMM is conventionally performed by reflux in ethanol, diphenyl ether, or toluene for 1–6 h at 100–160 °C, achieving to good yields (70–85%) (Scheme 2a) [18–20]. However, metal-catalyzed [5,21] reactions could provide better yields (>95%). Solvent-free microwave (MW)-assisted synthesis has also been developed and reported as an improved reaction and environmentally friendly approach to synthesizing DAMSs [22,23] (Scheme 2b), whose main advantages are related to the MW mediated reaction rate acceleration owing to the selective heating of more polar reactants by MW irradiation [24]. Thus, MW-assisted synthesis of DAMMs can offer short reaction times, excellent compatibility of various substituents, the absence of solvents and catalysts, low energy consumption, and high yields (>78%).

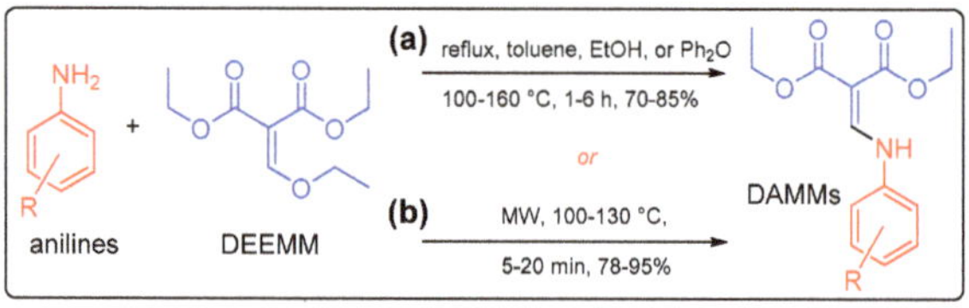

Scheme 2. Synthetic versions for the synthesis of diethyl 2-((arylamino)methylene)malonates (DAMMs) using the first step of the Gould-Jacobs reaction. (**a**) reflux-based protocol; (**b**) MW-assisted protocol. MW = microwave irradiation; DEEMM = diethyl ethoxymethylenemalonate.

Although DAMMs have mainly been employed as valuable intermediates for synthesizing biologically active compounds, and they are commercially available, their biological properties have not been deeply studied, even though they have shown bioactivity in certain studies [19]. In addition, they contain an enamine ester moiety which has been recognized to exhibit attractive antifungal activity in different enamine-containing compounds [25,26]. With observations of activity as evidenced by the above-mentioned DAMM-contaminated PS2Ps in mind, these structural features led us to hypothesize that DAMMs exhibit antifungal activity against *Fox*, constituting the main contribution and novelty of our study. In this regard, this paper is intended to report, for the first time, the antifungal activity of a small set of DAMMs, prepared through the reported, advantageous MW-assisted protocol. In this study, the DAMM products contained various representative substitutions, allowing us to explore their influence on antifungal activity preliminarily, through mycelial growth inhibition against *Fox*, and contributing to the discovery of bioactive compounds which may be particularly useful in the plant pathology field.

2. Results and Discussion

2.1. Synthesis of the DAMMs **1–5**

The target products were synthesized following the reported methodology (Scheme 3) to prepare DAMMs as intermediates, with some modifications [22]. This methodology has already been reported under the following reaction conditions: 115 °C (300 W) for 10 min. However, in our attempts with the available MW reactor, the reaction time and temperature were found to be different, i.e., 30 min and 150 °C (200 W), respectively. These variations resulted from a testing temperature ramp performed between 90–150 °C using DEEMM and *p*-chloroaniline as model reagents to afford DAMM **1** for comparative purposes (Scheme 3a). Under these conditions, the formation of **1** could be observed at 150 °C, whose TLC band was different from the starting reagents. The reaction was monitored by TLC every 5 min and, after 20 min, the expected product was formed, as revealed with iodine vapor, UV (254–366 nm), and Dragendorff's reagent. After 30 min, the reagents were entirely consumed, and the reaction was quenched. The resulting crude product was then purified by column chromatography (*n*-hexane/ethyl acetate 7:3) to afford isolated **1** (80% yield).

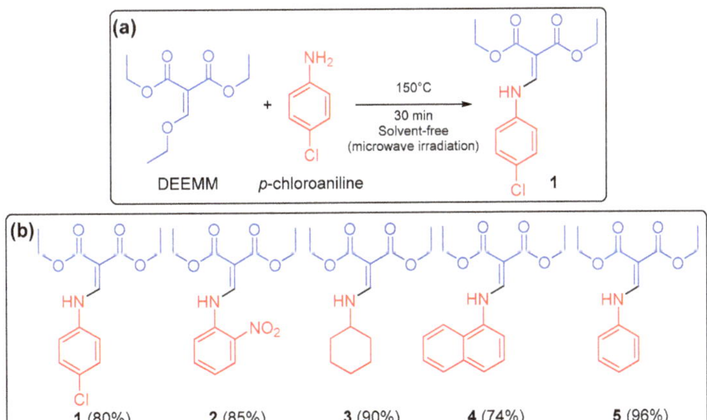

Scheme 3. (**a**). One-step reaction for the free-solvent synthesis of diethyl 2-(((4-chlorophenyl)amino) methylene)malonate (DAMM) **1** by a microwave-assisted procedure as the model reaction. (**b**). Structures of the synthesized DAMMs **1–5** and their reaction yield in parenthesis. DEEMM = diethyl ethoxymethylenemalonate.

This reported protocol, experimentally optimized to suit our laboratory conditions, was used to prepare additional DAMMs **2–5** by employing several primary amines containing representative moieties in order to examine their influence on the DAMM synthesis, i.e., *o*-nitrophenyl, cyclohexyl, 1-naphthyl, and phenyl, whose structures and yields are shown in Scheme 3b. Although some yield variations were identified between the five products, the outcome indicated good to excellent yields (74–96%). The results led us to briefly describe the influence of some precursor amines on the resulting yields. For instance, product **4**, containing a 1-naphthylamine (bulkier substituent), afforded a 74%

yield. This yield can be compared to that of **5**, which includes a phenylamine moiety as a less bulky substituent and afforded the highest yield (96%). Additionally, it was evidenced that the product prepared from aniline with an electron-withdrawing group (EWG) at the *ortho* position, e.g., **2** (85%), showed a similar yield to the product afforded from aniline with a weak EWG at the *para* position, e.g., **1** (80%). This reaction is also facilitated by using primary amines with an alicyclic substituent, e.g., cyclohexyl amine, which afforded product **3** in good yield (90%). The NMR data of compounds **1**, **2**, and **5** have already been reported in the literature [7,19]; however, in the case of compounds **3** and **4**, only chromatographic data can be found so far and, consequently, the present study provides such data (Supplementary Material).

2.2. *Antifungal Activity of DAMMs* **1–5**

As mentioned, our aim was based on the discovered antifungal effect of DAMMs when they were formed as side-products during a three-component domino reaction to produce PS2Ps. Thus, once the DAMM antifungal activity was noticed, we employed a known reaction to produce the desired compounds in convenient amounts to validate our previous findings related to the antifungal activity. Hence, DAMMs **1–5** were synthesized, isolated to high purity, and evaluated through an in vitro bioassay to assess their capacity to inhibit the mycelial growth of the phytopathogen *Fox* for 72 h. Five concentrations (between 10–0.01 μg/μL) of each test compound were employed for this procedure. Dithane (active ingredient: mancozeb) and Rovral (active ingredient: iprodione) were used as the positive controls, and PDA 0.5% was used as the blank. The antifungal activity results for compounds **1–5** are shown in Figure 1.

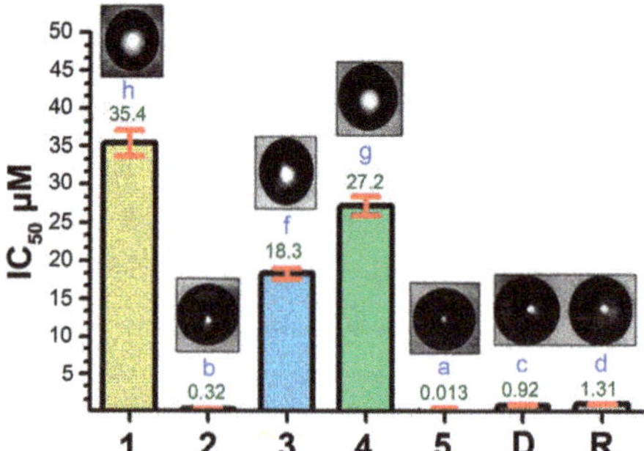

Figure 1. Antifungal activity against *F. oxysporum* (*Fox*) for the diethyl 2-((aryl(alkyl)amino) methylene)malonates **1–5** and positive controls (D: Dithane; R: Rovral). Green values over bars correspond to the mean half-maximal inhibitory concentrations (IC_{50} in μM), with red error bars representing the interval confidence. Different blue lowercase letters over bars indicate statistically significant differences according to the Tukey test ($p < 0.05$). Pictures over bars correspond to the observed fungistatic or fungicide effect on *Fox*.

The antifungal activity of DAMMs **1–5** followed a dose–response behavior to inhibit the mycelial growth of *Fox*. The best antifungal activity was obtained for **2** and **5** ($IC_{50} < 0.5$ μM), while **1**, **3**, and **4** were less active (18 μM < IC_{50} < 35 μM). The most active DAMM was compound **5**, whose activity was even better than those of the positive controls, constituting a promising antifungal activity against *Fox*. Due to compound **5** not having substitutions in the aromatic ring, and the least active DAMM being **1**, we concluded that the substituent evidenced an unfavorable impact on bioactivity in **1** (e.g., *p*-Cl). However, compound **2** also showed important antifungal activity against *Fusarium oxysporum*, since the IC_{50} was less than 1 μM, suggesting that the *ortho*-substituted nitro group may positively contribute to the inhibition of *Fox*. Likewise, compounds **4** and **3** (having 1-naphthyl and cyclohexyl, respectively, as *N*-substitution) showed low activity, suggesting that a bulky moiety and an aliphatic ring are plausibly related to the reduced antifungal activity of the tested DAMMs. These observations require further studies, expanding the DAMM chemical space and providing more insights into the structure-dependent variations of the antifungal activity. Additionally, the most-active compounds (**2** and **5**) and positive controls were classified as fungicides (i.e., fungus could not grow in fresh medium after exposure to these treatments), whereas compounds **1**, **3**, and **4** were found to exhibit a fungistatic effect. This fact is also favorable for compound **5** as a promising antifungal, since its effect on *Fox* mycelial growth inhibition was remarkable (IC_{50} = 13 nM), acting as a fungicide [27].

3. Materials and Methods

3.1. General

All starting reagents (primary amines and diethyl ethoxymethylenmalonate) were obtained commercially from Merck (Darmstadt, Germany) and Sigma-Aldrich (Burlington, MA, USA). The reactions were monitored by thin-layer chromatography (TLC) using Silica gel 60 F254. The mobile phase was 7:3 ethyl hexane-acetate, and Dragendorff's reagent, iodine vapors, UV-254 nm, and 366 nm were used as developers. For the separation and purification of the reaction crude, column chromatography (CC) was used as the stationary phase using Merck column silica (0.063–0.200 mm) and as the mobile phase a 7:3 *n*-hexane-ethyl acetate mixture. Additionally, preparative chromatography was used for purification using 0.5 mm thick PLC (preparative layer chromatography) glass chromatographic plates (Merck KGaA, Darmstadt, Germany) on which 100 μL of the reaction crude product was seeded and eluted in 50 mL of hexane-ethyl acetate 7:3 mixture as a mobile phase for 1 h. Subsequently, the plate was monitored by UV (254 nm), and the analyte surface to be separated was labeled. Once the silica/target compound mixture was removed from PLC plates, it was vacuum filtered in a Pyrex™ borosilicate glass funnel with a sintered glass disk and eluted with HPLC-grade methanol. Finally, the compound was concentrated in a rotary evaporator, stored in a clean, dry, and weighed container, and monitored by TLC to verify its purity. High-resolution mass spectrometry analyses with electrospray ionization (ESI) were performed using a Bruker micrOTOF–QII mass spectrometer, consisting of two analytical pumps (model LC-20AD) with SIL-20AHT automatic injector, SPD-20A UV/Vis detector, CTO-20A column oven, and CBM-20A controller. Each compound analyzed by this technique was prepared at 1 mg/mL using LCMS grade methanol as solvent. The column used was a Phenomenex Luna PFP (2) (5 μm, 150 × 2 mm). The flow was 0.2 mL/min, and the mobile phase comprised solvents A (0.1% formic acid in H_2O) and B (0.1% formic acid in MeOH). The employed gradient was 0 min, 5% B, maintained for 2 min, from 5 to 30 min until 100% B, and maintained 100% B for 25 min. The oven temperature was 40 °C, and the wavelength was 254 and 280 nm. The ESI interface was operated in a positive mode with 4.5 kV in the capillary and 0.5 kV in the endplate offset. The nebulization gas pressure was 0.4 Bar; the drying gas was maintained at a flow rate of 8 L/min at 200 °C. The collision and the quadrupole energy were set to 12 and 6 eV, respectively. RF1 and RF2 funnels were programmed to 150 and 200 Vpp, respectively. The mass spectra were calibrated using sodium formate. The results were processed in data analysis software to determine the accurate masses. The ^{1}H NMR spectra were recorded at 500 MHz on a spectrometer DRX 500 (Bruker, Billerica, MA, USA) using $CDCl_3$ as a solvent and tetramethylsilane (TMS, 0.05% *v*/*v*) as an internal standard (TMS δ 0.00). Each spectrum resulted from 128 scans with pulse widths (PW) of 8.0 μs (30 °C) and relaxation delays (RD) of 6.0 s. Chemical shifts were expressed in δ (ppm) involving solvent signals at δ_H 7.26 and δ_C 77.16. Multiplicities were abbreviated as follows: singlet (*s*), doublet (*d*), triplet (*t*), quartet (*q*), and multiplet (*m*). The coupling constants (*J*) were expressed in Hz.

3.2. General Procedure for the Microwave-Assisted Synthesis of Diethyl 2-((aryl(alkyl)amino) methylene)malonates **1–5**

The general procedure to synthesize DAMMs was adopted from a reported protocol [22] with some modifications. Briefly, diethyl ethoxymethylenemalonate (1.0 mmol)

(Sigma-Aldrich, Burlington, MA, USA) and primary amines (0.5 mmol) were placed into a 5.0 mL high-pressure reaction tube. The tube was closed and stirred for 1 h at room temperature to mix the raw materials well. Subsequently, the reaction mixture was placed in a CEM brand Discover SP microwave synthesizer (CEM, Matthews, NC, USA) for 30 min at 150 °C. Then, the reaction crude product was monitored by TLC using an *n*-hexane-ethyl acetate mobile phase (7:3 ratio), followed by purification by column chromatography and/or preparative plate chromatography. Finally, the products were revealed with Dragendorff's reagent, showing red bands as a positive test for nitrogen-containing compounds. The MS and NMR spectra and spectroscopical data of compounds **1–5** are provided in the Supplementary Material.

3.3. Antifungal Activity

Antifungal activity evaluation of diethyl 2-((aryl(alkyl)amino)methylene)malonates **1–5** was performed by measuring the growth halo of the phytopathogen *F. oxysporum* in the presence of the test compounds at different concentrations compared to a blank (PDA 0.5% without treatment). The culture medium contained 2.4% PDB and 1.5% bacteriological agar in 100 mL of distilled water. First, the medium was homogenized for 2 min in a microwave oven and then sterilized in an autoclave for 1 h at 120 °C. Next, 20 mL of the sterile medium was placed in a sterilized Petri dish. Once it cooled and solidified, a 2-mm plug from a previously prepared monosporic culture was placed onto the central part of the Petri dish and left to grow at 28 °C for 8 days to propagate the fungus.

This antifungal assay involved five concentrations (10, 5, 1, 0.1, and 0.01 µg/µL) of test diethyl 2-((aryl(alkyl)amino)methylene)malonates **1–5** as treatments. They were dispersed in a 0.5% supplemented medium [28]. Subsequently, each treatment was randomly placed into a well of a 12-well glass plate (79 × 63 × 4 mm). Finally, a 1-mm plug from the 8-day fungal monosporic culture with a diameter proportional to a 32-mm borosilicate capillary tube was taken and placed onto the central part of each well containing a dispersed treatment into the medium. The plate was placed in a humid chamber for 72 h at 25 °C. The assessment of each concentration per treatment was performed in triplicate. After incubation, a photograph of the 12-well plate was taken and analyzed in ImageJ software. The growth area was then measured. The measured growth areas were employed to calculate the inhibition percentage compared to the blank as follows: % Inhibition = ((blank growth area–target compound growth area)/blank growth area). The calculated inhibition percentages per concentration were used to build a dose–response curve, and the half maximal inhibitory concentration was calculated by nonlinear regression in Graph Pad Prism 5.0 software.

3.3.1. Fungicidal and Fungistatic Effect

For the fungicidal or fungistatic activity classification procedure, the central plug of the fungus treated with the highest concentration (10 µg/µL) of each test compound **1–5** was placed on a fresh, non-amended PDA medium for 72 h. After this, mycelial growth was further monitored. The diethyl 2-((aryl(alkyl)amino)methylene)malonates **1–5** were classified as fungistatic or fungicidal if mycelial growth or no mycelial growth, respectively was observed [29].

3.3.2. Statistical Analysis

A Shapiro-Wilks normality test was performed to assess the normal distribution of the data ($p > 0.05$). Once normal data distribution had been verified, an analysis of variance (ANOVA) was carried out, followed by a post hoc Tukey test to establish significant differences between treatments ($p < 0.05$). These analyses were performed in Infostat statistical software [30].

4. Conclusions

A small set of diethyl 2-((aryl(alkyl)amino)methylene)malonates (**1–5**), i.e., side-products of a PS2P-producing domino reaction and prepared by an MW-assisted protocol (>74% yield), showed antifungal activity at different levels. The resulting IC_{50} values of test compounds ranged from 0.013 to 35 μM. The best antifungal outcome was obtained for the test DAMMs with an *ortho*-nitro-substituted or non-substituted aromatic ring (i.e., **2** and **5**, respectively). These two antifungal DAMMs were classified as fungicidal agents, having a promising mycelial growth inhibition effect at the nanomolar scale (320 and 13 nM, respectively). Therefore, they can be considered active candidates for fungicide development to be helpful in plant disease management by controlling the economically relevant phytopathogen, *Fox*.

Supplementary Materials: The following supporting information can be downloaded online, Physical and spectroscopical data of DAMMs (**1–5**); Figure S1: High-resolution mass spectra of compound **1**; Figure S2: Assignments of ^{1}H and ^{13}C NMR chemical shifts of compound **1**; Figure S3: ^{1}H NMR spectrum ($CDCl_3$, 500 MHz) of compound **1**; Figure S4: ^{13}C NMR spectrum ($CDCl_3$, 125 MHz) of compound **1**; Figure S5: High-resolution mass spectra of compound **2**; Figure S6: Assignments of ^{1}H and ^{13}C NMR chemical shifts of compound **2**; Figure S7: ^{1}H NMR spectrum ($CDCl_3$, 500 MHz) of compound **2**; Figure S8: ^{13}C NMR spectrum ($CDCl_3$, 125 MHz) of compound **2**; Figure S9: High-resolution mass spectra of compound **3**; Figure S10: Assignments of ^{1}H and ^{13}C NMR chemical shifts of compound **3**; Figure S11: ^{1}H NMR spectrum ($CDCl_3$, 500 MHz) of compound **3**; Figure S12: ^{13}C NMR spectrum ($CDCl_3$, 125 MHz) of compound **3**; Figure S13: High-resolution mass spectra of compound **4**; Figure S14: Assignments of ^{1}H and ^{13}C NMR chemical shifts of compound **4**; Figure S15: ^{1}H NMR spectrum ($CDCl_3$, 500 MHz) of compound **4**; Figure S16: ^{13}C NMR spectrum ($CDCl_3$, 125 MHz) of compound **4**; Figure S17: High-resolution mass spectra of compound **5**; Figure S18: Assignments of ^{1}H and ^{13}C NMR chemical shifts of compound **5**; Figure S19: ^{1}H NMR spectrum ($CDCl_3$, 500 MHz) of compound **5**; Figure S20: ^{13}C NMR spectrum ($CDCl_3$, 125 MHz) of compound **5**; Scheme S1. Reaction mechanism to produce DAMMs.

Author Contributions: Conceptualization, E.C.-B.; methodology, W.-F.C.-V.; software, W.-F.C.-V. and E.C.-B.; validation, W.-F.C.-V., D.Q. and E.C.-B.; formal analysis, W.-F.C.-V. and E.C.-B.; resources, D.Q. and E.C.-B.; data curation, W.-F.C.-V. and E.C.-B.; writing—original draft preparation, W.-F.C.-V.; writing—review and editing, W.-F.C.-V., D.Q. and E.C.-B.; supervision, E.C.-B.; project administration, E.C.-B.; funding acquisition, D.Q. and E.C.-B. All authors have read and agreed to the published version of the manuscript.

Funding: This study was funded by Universidad Militar Nueva Granada (UMNG), grant number IMP-CIAS-2924, validity 2020.

Institutional Review Board Statement: Not applicable.

Informed Consent Statement: Not applicable.

Data Availability Statement: The data presented in this study are available from the corresponding author upon reasonable request.

Acknowledgments: The authors thank the UMNG for the financial support.

Conflicts of Interest: The authors declare no conflict of interest.

Appendix A

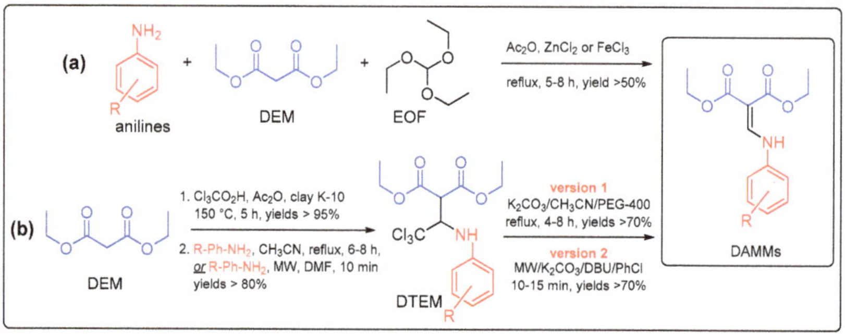

Scheme A1. Synthetic strategies for the synthesis of diethyl 2-((arylamino)methylene)malonates (DAMMs). (**a**) multicomponent strategy; (**b**) three-step strategy. DEM = Diethyl malonate; EOF = ethyl orthoformate; MW = microwave irradiation; DTEM = 2-(2,2,2-trifluoro-1-(phenylamino) ethyl)malonate; DMF = *N*,*N*-dimethylformamide; PEG-400 = polyethylenglycol-400; DBU = 1,8-diazabicyclo(5.4.0)undec-7-ene.

References

1. Hu, M.; Chen, S. Non-Target Site Mechanisms of Fungicide Resistance in Crop Pathogens: A Review. *Microorganisms* **2021**, *9*, 502. [CrossRef] [PubMed]
2. Al-Hatmi, A.M.; de Hoog, G.S.; Meis, J.F. Multiresistant Fusarium Pathogens on Plants and Humans: Solutions in (from) the Antifungal Pipeline? *Infect. Drug Resist.* **2019**, *12*, 3727–3737. [CrossRef] [PubMed]
3. Bai, H.; Sun, R.; Chen, X.; Yang, L.; Huang, C. Microwave-Assisted, Solvent-Free, Three-Component Domino Protocol: Efficient Synthesis of Polysubstituted-2-Pyridone Derivatives. *ChemistrySelect* **2018**, *3*, 4635–4638. [CrossRef]
4. Larson, P.G.; Ferguson, D.M. 4-Amino-2-Butyl-7-Methoxycarbonylthiazolo[4,5-c]Quinoline. *Molbank* **2021**, *2021*, 1305. [CrossRef]
5. Banerji, B.; Conejo-Garcia, A.; McNeill, L.A.; McDonough, M.A.; Buck, M.R.G.; Hewitson, K.S.; Oldham, N.J.; Schofield, C.J. The Inhibition of Factor Inhibiting Hypoxia-Inducible Factor (FIH) by β-Oxocarboxylic Acids. *Chem. Commun.* **2005**, *43*, 5438–5440. [CrossRef]
6. Ilangovan, A.; Kumar, R.G. 2,2-Bis(Ethoxycarbonyl)Vinyl (BECV) as a Versatile Amine Protecting Group for Selective Functional-Group Transformations. *Chem.–Eur. J.* **2010**, *16*, 2938–2943. [CrossRef]
7. Forezi, L.D.S.M.; Tolentino, N.M.C.; De Souza, A.M.T.; Castro, H.C.; Montenegro, R.C.; Dantas, R.F.; Oliveira, M.E.I.M.; Silva, F.P.; Barreto, L.H.; Burbano, R.M.R.; et al. Synthesis, Cytotoxicity and Mechanistic Evaluation of 4-Oxoquinoline-3- Carboxamide Derivatives: Finding New Potential Anticancer Drugs. *Molecules* **2014**, *19*, 6651–6670. [CrossRef]
8. Venkatesan, P.; Thamotharan, S.; Percino, M.J.; Ilangovan, A. Intramolecular Resonance Assisted N–H···O=C Hydrogen Bond and Weak Noncovalent Interactions in Two Asymmetrically Substituted Geminal Amido-Esters: Crystal Structures and Quantum Chemical Exploration. *J. Mol. Struct.* **2021**, *1246*, 131210. [CrossRef]
9. Deshmukh, A.R.A.S.; Panse, D.G.; Bhawal, B.M. A Clay Catalyzed Method for Diethyl 2,2,2- Trichloroethylidenepropanedioate, an Efficient Intermediate for the Synthesis of Enamino Esters. *Synth. Commun.* **1999**, *29*, 1801–1809. [CrossRef]
10. Ilangovan, A.; Kumar, R.; Kaushik, M. Lewis Acid Mediated Selective Monohydrolysis of Geminal Diesters: Synthesis of Functionalized Malonic Acid Half Esters. *Synlett* **2012**, *23*, 2093–2097. [CrossRef]
11. Arya, F.; Bouquant, J.; Chuche, J. A Convenient Synthesis of 3-Formyl-4(1 h)-Pyridones. *Synthesis (Stuttgart)* **1983**, *1983*, 946–948. [CrossRef]
12. Tsoung, J.; Bogdan, A.R.; Kantor, S.; Wang, Y.; Charaschanya, M.; Djuric, S.W. Synthesis of Fused Pyrimidinone and Quinolone Derivatives in an Automated Hight-Temperature and High-Pressure Flow Reactor. *J. Org. Chem.* **2017**, *82*, 1073–1084. [CrossRef]
13. Muñoz, H.; Tamariz, J.; Zamora, H.S.; Lázaro, M.; Labarrios, F. Preparation of Propanedioic Acid, (Anilinometwlene) Alkyl Esters by Direct Condensation. *Synth. Commun.* **1987**, *17*, 549–554. [CrossRef]
14. Bhujanga Rao, A.K.S.; Radhakrishna, A.S.; Rao, C.G.; Singh, B.B.; Bhatnagar, S.P. An Improved Procedure for the Preparation of Ethyl α-Carbethoxy-β-(Arylamino)Acrylates. *Org. Prep. Proced. Int.* **1988**, *20*, 93–95. [CrossRef]
15. Wang, Z. Gould-Jacobs Reaction. In *Comprehensive Organic Name Reactions and Reagents*; Wang, Z., Ed.; John Wiley & Sons, Inc.: Hoboken, NJ, USA, 2010; pp. 1252–1255, ISBN 9780470638859.
16. Li, J.J. Gould–Jacobs Reaction. In *Name Reactions: A Collection of Detailed Mechanisms and Synthetic Applications*; Li, J.J., Ed.; Springer International Publishing: Berlin/Heidelberg, Germany, 2014; pp. 289–290, ISBN 978-3-319-03979-4.
17. Loupy, A.; Song, S.J.; Cho, S.J.; Park, D.K.; Kwon, T.W. Solvent-free Microwave Michael Addition between EMME and Various Nucleophiles. *Synth. Commun.* **2005**, *35*, 79–87. [CrossRef]

8. Lager, E.; Andersson, P.; Nilsson, J.; Pettersson, I.; Nielsen, E.Ø.; Nielsen, M.; Sterner, O.; Liljefors, T. 4-Quinolone Derivatives: High-Affinity Ligands at the Benzodiazepine Site of Brain GABAA Receptors. Synthesis, Pharmacology, and Pharmacophore Modeling. *J. Med. Chem.* **2006**, *49*, 2526–2533. [CrossRef]
9. Shaik, A.; Angira, D.; Thiruvenkatam, V. Insights into Supramolecular Assembly Formation of Diethyl Aryl Amino Methylene Malonate (DAM)Derivatives Assisted via Non-Covalent Interactions. *J. Mol. Struct.* **2019**, *1192*, 178–185. [CrossRef]
0. Santos, C.; Pimentel, L.; Canzian, H.; Oliveira, A.; Junior, F.; Dantas, R.; Hoelz, L.; Marinho, D.; Cunha, A.; Bastos, M.; et al. Hybrids of Imatinib with Quinoline: Synthesis, Antimyeloproliferative Activity Evaluation, and Molecular Docking. *Pharmaceuticals* **2022**, *15*, 309. [CrossRef]
1. Jang, T.-S.; Ku, I.W.; Jang, M.S.; Keum, G.; Kang, S.B.; Chung, B.Y.; Kim, Y. Indium-Mediated One-Pot Three-Component Reaction of Aromatic Amines, Enol Ethers, and Allylic Bromides. *Org. Lett.* **2006**, *8*, 195–198. [CrossRef]
2. Malvacio, I.; Vera, D.; Moyano, E. Microwave Assisted Synthesis of Ethyl-Quinolon-4-One-3-Carboxylates and Hydrolysis to Quinolon-4-One-3-Carboxylic Acids. *Curr. Microw. Chem.* **2014**, *1*, 52–58. [CrossRef]
3. Cernuchová, P.; Vo-Thanh, G.; Milata, V.; Loupy, A. Solvent-Free Synthesis of Quinolone Derivatives. *Heterocycles* **2004**, *64*, 177–191. [CrossRef]
4. Li, X.; Xu, J. Determination on Temperature Gradient of Different Polar Reactants in Reaction Mixture under Microwave Irradiation with Molecular Probe. *Tetrahedron* **2016**, *72*, 5515–5520. [CrossRef]
5. Borrego-Muñoz, P.; Cardenas, D.; Ospina, F.; Coy-Barrera, E.; Quiroga, D. Second-Generation Enamine-Type Schiff Bases as 2-Amino Acid-Derived Antifungals against Fusarium Oxysporum: Microwave-Assisted Synthesis, in Vitro Activity, 3D-QSAR, and in Vivo Effect. *J. Fungi* **2023**, *9*, 113. [CrossRef] [PubMed]
6. Borrego-Muñoz, P.; Becerra, L.D.; Ospina, F.; Coy-Barrera, E.; Quiroga, D. Synthesis (Z) vs (E) Selectivity, Antifungal Activity against Fusarium Oxysporum, and Structure-Based Virtual Screening of Novel Schiff Bases Derived from L-Tryptophan. *ACS Omega* **2022**, *7*, 24714–24726. [CrossRef]
7. Ul Haq, I.; Sarwar, M.K.; Faraz, A.; Latif, M.Z. Synthetic Chemicals: Major Component of Plant Disease Management. In *Plant Disease Management Strategies for Sustainable Agriculture through Traditional and Modern Approaches*; Ul Haq, I., Ijaz, S., Eds.; Springer International Publishing: Cham, Switzerland, 2020; pp. 53–81, ISBN 978-3-030-35955-3.
8. Marentes-Culma, R.; Orduz-Díaz, L.L.; Coy-Barrera, E. Targeted Metabolite Profiling-Based Identification of Antifungal 5-*n*-Alkylresorcinols Occurring in Different Cereals against *Fusarium oxysporum*. *Molecules* **2019**, *24*, 770. [CrossRef]
9. Cole, M.D. Key Antifungal, Antibacterial and Anti-Insect Assays-a Critical Review. *Biochem. Syst. Ecol.* **1994**, *22*, 837–856. [CrossRef]
0. Di Rienzo, J.A.; Casanoves, F.; Balzarini, M.G.; Gonzalez, L.; Tablada, M.; Robledo, C.W. *InfoStat*; versión 24; Universidad Nacional de Córdoba: Córdoba, Argentina, 2011; Available online: http://www.infostat.com.ar/ (accessed on 12 January 2023).

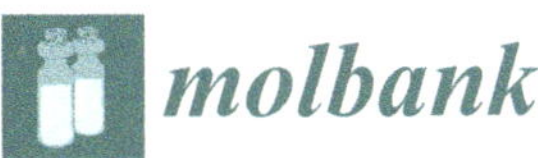 *molbank*

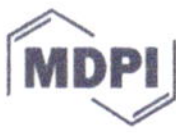

Short Note

4-(4-Ethoxyphenyl)-5-(4-methoxyphenyl)-2,4-dihydro-3*H*-1,2,4-triazol-3-one

Ion Burcă [1], Valentin Badea [1,*], Calin Deleanu [2,3], Vasile-Nicolae Bercean [1] and Francisc Péter [1]

1 Department of Applied Chemistry and Organic and Natural Compounds Engineering, Politehnica, University Timisoara, Carol Telbisz 6, 300001 Timisoara, Romania
2 "C. D. Nenitescu" Institute of Organic and Supramolecular Chemistry, Romanian Academy, Spl. Independentei 202B, 060023 Bucharest, Romania
3 "Petru Poni" Institute of Macromolecular Chemistry, Romanian Academy, Aleea Grigore Ghica Voda 41A, 700487 Iasi, Romania
* Correspondence: valentin.badea@upt.ro; Tel.: +40-742-044-969

Abstract: A new triazol-3-one resulted unexpectedly from the reduction reaction of a heterocyclic thioketone using sodium borohydride in pyridine containing a small amount of water. The structure of the new compound was characterised using FT-IR, 1D and 2D NMR, and HRMS spectroscopic methods.

Keywords: triazol-3-one; reduction; heterocyclic ketone; S-alkylation

1. Introduction

Triazoles are a class of five-membered heterocycles that contain three nitrogen and two carbon atoms. On the basis of the way nitrogen and carbon atoms connect between each other, there exist two triazole isomers: 1,2,3-triazoles and 1,2,4-triazoles. These compounds have been extensively studied for more than a century due to their remarkable properties, making them promising candidates for drug development and treatment of various diseases [1]. Some of the most known drugs that contain the 1,2,4-triazole moiety are alprazolam, fluconazole, ribavirin, and posaconazole.

1,2,4-triazoles that contain the sulphanyl functional group directly attached to the heterocyclic core have also been studied for their potential use as bioactive compounds. The first reported synthesis of 3-sulphanyl-1,2,4-triazole was reported by Freund in 1896 [2]. Some of the biological activities of 1,2,4-triazole thiols include anticancer [3,4], enzyme inhibition capacity [5], antioxidant [6], antimicrobial [7], anti-inflammatory [8], antituberculous [9], and many more.

Several methods are commonly used to synthesise 3-sulphanyl-1,2,4-triazoles, including reactions involving the reaction of isothiocyanates with hydrazides [10] and the reaction of 1,3,4-oxadiazoles with hydrazine [11], by thermal cyclization of acylated thiosemicarbazides [12] or by reaction between carboxylic acids with hydrazinecarbothiohydrazides [13].

S-alkylated compounds can be prepared by reacting the corresponding sulphanyl compound with a halogenated compound under various reaction conditions. Some of the reported S-alkylation protocols include the use of potassium carbonate [14], potassium hydroxide [15], caesium carbonate [16], sodium ethoxide [17], and ultrasound [18].

1,2,4-triazole-3-ones are heterocyclic compounds that have biological activities such as anticonvulsant [19], anti-inflammatory [20], and antimicrobial [21,22]. In addition, these compounds can be used as high-energy materials [23].

Taking into account the aforementioned information, our aim was to synthesise novel sulphanyl-alkylated 1,2,4-triazoles. During an intermediate synthesis step, an unexpected outcome occurred when the carbonyl intermediate was reduced using sodium borohydride, leading to the formation of a triazolone through a new, unreported method.

Citation: Burcă, I.; Badea, V.; Deleanu, C.; Bercean, V.-N.; Péter, F. 4-(4-Ethoxyphenyl)-5-(4-methoxyphenyl)-2,4-dihydro-3*H*-1,2,4-triazol-3-one. *Molbank* **2023**, *2023*, M1705. https://doi.org/10.3390/M1705

Academic Editor: Stefano D'Errico

Received: 6 July 2023
Revised: 20 July 2023
Accepted: 25 July 2023
Published: 1 August 2023

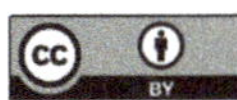

2. Results and Discussion

2-((4-(4-Ethoxyphenyl)-5-(4-methoxyphenyl)-4*H*-1,2,4-triazol-3-yl)thio)-1-phenylethan-1-one **(2)** was synthesized using an S-alkylation reaction of the 4-(4-ethoxyphenyl)-5-(4-methoxyphenyl)-4*H*-1,2,4-triazole-3-thiol **(1)**. Initially, the scope of the present work was to synthesise a secondary racemic alcohol from the aforementioned ketone by reduction of carbonylic functional group using sodium borohydride. Therefore, a modified procedure from the literature was applied for the reduction reaction. The synthesis followed Scheme 1:

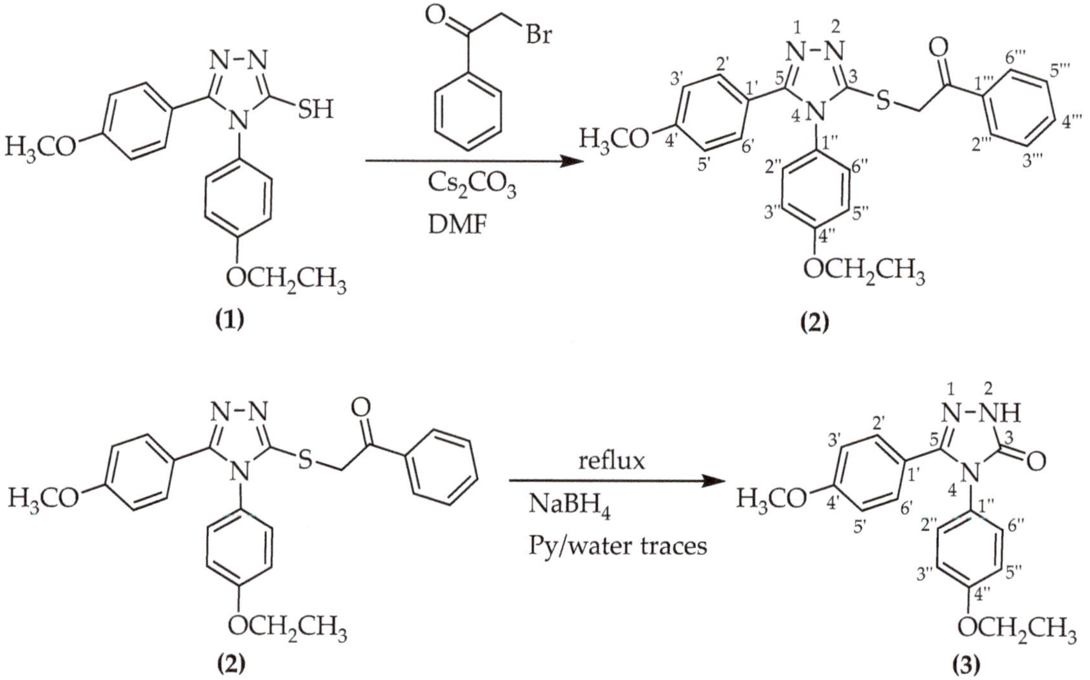

Scheme 1. Synthesis scheme for the novel compound **(3)**.

For the S-alkylation reaction, a modified reported protocol was followed [16]. The caesium carbonate was used in excess in relation to triazole thiol. As an alkylation agent, 2-bromo-1-phenylethan-1-one was used. During the reaction, in the basic medium provided by caesium carbonate, an intermediate thiolate salt is formed. Due to the conjugation of the triazole ring and the presence of the sulphur atom with its lone pair of electrons, the salt possesses a nucleophilic character, so it readily reacts with the α-haloketone. In addition to the aromatic and ether functional groups, the resulting compound carries a ketone and thioether functional group. Like other carbonylic compounds, it can be reduced to an alcohol by using different reduction agents.

For the reduction of the obtained ketone, sodium borohydride was chosen as the reduction agent, following modified literature procedures [24]. An excess of the borohydride was used to compensate for the eventual loss of reduction agent by decomposition or secondary reactions. Surprisingly, the reduction reaction did not produce racemic secondary alcohol, but rather a different compound **(3)**. First, it possessed an unusually high melting point, which is not characteristic of similar secondary racemic alcohols. From NMR and later HRMS data, it was concluded that the obtained compound carries a ketone functional group but it is directly attached to the triazole ring. At first sight, it appears that the reaction of heterocyclic thioketones with sodium borohydride in the pyridine/water mixture at reflux temperature leads to the formation of triazolone **(3)** instead of the secondary alcohol. A first conclusion is that instead of the reduction of carbonyl group, a nucleophilic substitution of the alkylsulphanyl functional group by the hydroxyl functional group in the basic medium took place. More research in this direction is required to elucidate the real mechanism of the reaction. It is not clear what effect the alkyl substituents or reaction conditions (temperature, solvent, etc.) have on the triazolone formation rate. In Scheme 2, the expected and actual reaction paths are represented.

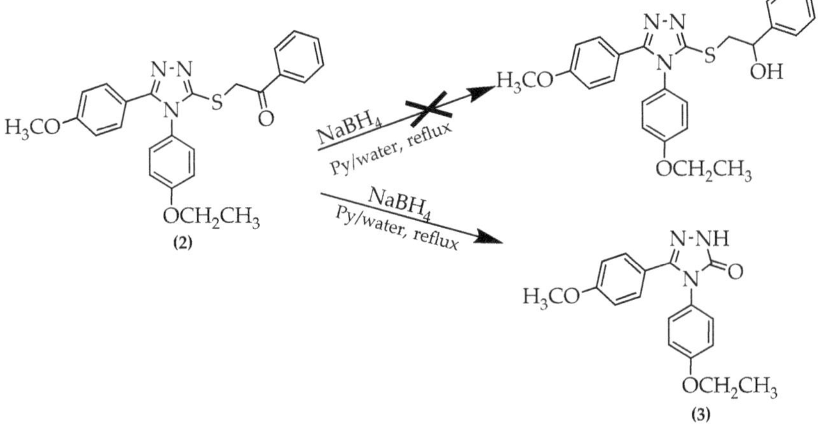

Scheme 2. Unexpected formation of **(3)** by reduction of compound **(2)**.

2.1. *Explanation of Experimental NMR Data for Compound* (2)

From the ^{1}H-^{15}N HMBC spectrum, the signals corresponding to aromatic protons 2″-H and 6″-H (7.16 ppm) were identified by the long-range coupling with 4-N nitrogen atom (174.9 ppm). In the ^{1}H-^{13}C HMBC spectrum, the following long-range couplings could be observed: coupling of the carbonylic carbon (C=O) (193.3 ppm) with aromatic protons 2‴-H and 6‴-H (8.04 ppm), coupling of carbon atom 3-C (152.2 ppm) with methylene protons (S-CH_2) (4.95 ppm), coupling of carbon atom 5-C (155.1 ppm) with aromatic protons 2′-H and 6′-H (7.36 ppm), coupling of carbon atom 4′-C (160.6 ppm) with methyl protons (O-CH_3) (3.77 ppm), and the coupling of carbon atom 4″-C (159.9 ppm) with methylene protons (O-CH_2) (4.07 ppm). In Table 1, long-range correlations between protons and carbon atoms (^{1}H-^{13}C HMBC experiment) and long-range correlation between protons and nitrogen atom (^{1}H-^{15}N HMBC) are presented.

Table 1. Experimental NMR data * for the compound **(2)**.

HMBC (^{1}H-^{15}N)	HMBC (^{1}H-^{13}C)
174.9 → 7.16 (4-N) (2″-H, 6″-H)	193.3 → 8.04 (C = O) (2‴-H, 6‴-H) 152.2 → 4.95 (3-C) (S-CH_2) 155.1 → 7.36 (5-C) (2′-H, 6′-H) 160.6 → 3.77 (4′-C) (O-CH_3) 159.9 → 4.07 (4″-C) (O-CH_2)

*—The values of the chemical shifts are given in ppm.

2.2. *Explanation of Experimental NMR Data for Compound* **(3)**

Using 2D NMR data, we could assign signals to all three nitrogen atoms of 1,2,4-triazole heterocycle as follows: from the ^{1}H-^{15}N HSQC spectrum, the direct coupling between nitrogen atom 2-N (164.5 ppm) and the directly attached proton 2-H (11.98 ppm). In the ^{1}H-^{15}N HMBC spectrum, long-range couplings between nitrogen atoms 4-N (154.1 ppm) and 1-N (254.5 ppm) and the proton 2-H (11.98 ppm) could be observed. The chemical shift identification of the nitrogen atom 4-N was performed based on its coupling with two aromatic protons 2″-H and 6″-H (7.16 ppm). In the long-range coupling spectrum ^{1}H-^{13}C HMBC, the couplings of the two triazolic carbon atoms 5-C (145.8 ppm) and 3-C (155.3 ppm) with the triazolic proton 2-H (11.98 ppm) were observed. The signal at 145.8 ppm was assigned to the 5-C carbon atom due to the couplings with aromatic protons 2′-H and 6′-H (7.22 ppm). The signals corresponding to 4′-C carbon (160.6 ppm) and 4″-C carbon (158.7 ppm) atoms were assigned based on the long-range couplings with methyl protons (O-CH_3) (3.72 ppm) and with methylene protons (O-CH_2) (4.03 ppm). In Table 2, direct bonding of protons to nitrogen atoms (^{1}H-^{15}N HSQC experiment), long-range correlations between protons and carbon atoms (^{1}H-^{13}C HMBC experiment), and long-range correlation between protons and nitrogen atom (^{1}H-^{15}N HMBC) are presented.

Table 2. Experimental NMR data * for the compound **(3)**.

HSQC (^{1}H-^{15}N)	**HMBC (^{1}H-^{15}N)**	**HMBC (^{1}H-^{13}C)**
164.4 → 11.98 (2-N) (2-H)	154.1 → 11.98 (4-N) (2-H)	145.8 → 11.98 (5-C) (2-H)
	254.5 → 11.98 (1-N) (2-H)	155.3 → 11.98 (3-C) (2-H)
	154.1 → 7.16 (4-N) (2″-H, 6″-H)	145.8 → 7.22 (5-C) (2′-H, 6′-H)
		160.6 → 3.72 (4′-C) (O-CH_3)
		158.7 → 4.03 (4″-C) (O-CH_2)

*—The values of the chemical shifts are given in ppm.

3. Materials and Methods

The reagents used were purchased from commercial sources and used as received. 4-(4-ethoxyphenyl)-5-(4-methoxyphenyl)-4*H*-1,2,4-triazole-3-thiol **(1)** was synthesized earlier in our laboratory following the modified procedures from the literature [25–27].

The ^{1}H-NMR, ^{13}C-NMR, and ^{15}N NMR spectra were recorded on a Bruker Avance III 500 MHz spectrometer. Chemical shifts (δ) have been measured in ppm and coupling constants (*J*) in Hz. The samples were dissolved in DMSO-*d6* or $CDCl_3$. TMS was used as an internal standard.

IR spectra were recorded on a Jasco FT/IR-410 spectrophotometer (Jasco Corporation, Tokyo, Japan) in KBr pellets.

Melting points were measured on a Böetius PHMK apparatus (Veb Analytik, Dresden) and were uncorrected.

The high-resolution MS (HRMS) spectrum was recorded on a Bruker Maxis II QTOF spectrometer (Bruker Daltonics, Bremen, Germany) with electrospray ionisation (ESI) in positive mode. The compound was initially dissolved in DMSO and further diluted 1:100 with acetonitrile. MS spectrum processing and isotope pattern simulations have been performed with Compass Data Analysis V.4.4 (Bruker Daltonics).

4. Experimental

4.1. Synthesis of 2-((4-(4-Ethoxyphenyl)-5-(4-methoxyphenyl)-4H-1,2,4-triazol-3-yl)thio)-1-phenylethan-1-one (2)

In a 100 mL round bottom flask equipped with a magnetic stirrer, 4-(4-ethoxyphenyl)-5-(4-methoxyphenyl)-4*H*-1,2,4-triazole-3-thiol (1 g, 3 mmol) was added together with 20 mL of DMF.

After complete dissolution of triazole-3-thiol **(1)**, caesium carbonate (0.992 g, 3 mmol) was added to the solution. A white precipitate formation was observed. The solution was stirred for 1 h to ensure that the whole triazole-3-thiol quantity was transformed into caesium 4-(4-ethoxyphenyl)-5-(4-methoxyphenyl)-4*H*-1,2,4-triazole-3-thiolate salt.

A solution of 2-bromo-1-phenylethan-1-one (0.642 g, 3.2 mmol) was prepared in 10 mL of 96% ethanol. Then, the obtained solution was added dropwise to the caesium thiolate salt under stirring. A slightly pink colouration of the solution was observed. After adding 2-bromo-1-phenylethan-1-one, the reaction mass was left to stir for 24 h. Reaction completion was monitored using TLC, using a 1:1 (*v/v*) hexane:ethyl acetate mixture as an eluent.

After 24 h, a white precipitate was observed in reaction mass, whereas the colour of the solution changed to a bright yellow one. The reaction mass was added dropwise to 150 mL of distilled water under vigorous stirring. A white precipitate was separated using vacuum filtration. After separation, the precipitate was dried at room temperature.

The precipitate was recrystallised from 35 mL of 96% ethanol.

920 mg of compound was obtained, and the isolation yield was 68%, melting point: 163–165 °C; ^{1}H NMR ($CDCl_3$, 500 MHz) δ (ppm): 8.04 (d, 2H, *J* = *7.2 Hz*, 2‴-H, 6‴-H), 7.62–7.58 (m, 1H, 4‴-H), 7.50–7.47 (m, 2H, 3‴-H, 5‴-H), 7.36 (d, 2H, *J* = *8.9 Hz*, 2′-H, 6′-H), 7.16 (d, 2H, *J* = *8.7 Hz*, 2″-H, 6″-H), 6.95 (d, 2H, *J* = *8.7 Hz*, 3″-H, 5″-H), 6.79 (d, 2H, *J* = *8.9Hz*, 3′-H, 5′-H), 4.95 (s, 2H, -S-CH_2-), 4.07 (q, 2H, -CH_2-CH_3), 3.77 (s, 3H, -CH_3), 1.45 (t, 3H, -CH_2-CH_3); ^{13}C NMR ($CDCl_3$, 125 MHz) δ (ppm): 193.3 (-C=O), 160.6 (4′-C), 159.9 (4″-C), 155.1 (5-C), 152.2 (3-C), 135.3 (1‴-C), 133.8 (4‴-C), 129.5 (2′-C, 6′-C), 128.8 (3‴, 5‴-C), 128.6 (2‴-C, 6‴-C), 128.5 (2″-C, 6″-C), 126.4 (4″-C), 119.1 (1′-C), 115.6 (2″-C, 6″-C), 113.9 (3′-C, 5′-C), 63.9 (-CH_2-CH_3), 59.2 (-CH_3), 41.1 (-S-CH_2), 14.7 (-CH_2-CH_3); ^{15}N NMR ($CDCl_3$, 50 MHz) δ (ppm): 174.9 (4-N); FT-IR (cm^{-1}): 3046 ($\nu_{Car\text{-}H}$), 3008 ($\nu_{Car\text{-}H}$), 2951 (ν^{as}_{CH3}), 2933 (ν^{as}_{CH3}), 1679 ($\nu_{C=O}$), 1609 ($\nu_{C=N\ triazole}$), 1578 ($\nu_{sk.ar.}$), 1510 ($\nu_{sk.ar.}$), 1479 ($\nu_{sk.ar.}$), 1254 (ν^{as}_{COC}).

4.2. Synthesis of 4-(4-Ethoxyphenyl)-5-(4-methoxyphenyl)-2,4-dihydro-3H-1,2,4-triazol-3-one (3)

In a 100 mL round bottom flask equipped with a magnetic stirrer, 2-((4-(4-ethoxyphenyl)-5-(4-methoxyphenyl)-4*H*-1,2,4-triazol-3-yl)thio)-1-phenylethan-1-one (0.72 g, 2 mmol) was added to 10 mL of pyridine and 1 mL of distilled water, then the heating of the reaction mixture with stirring was started.

During 30 min, small portions of sodium borohydride (0.302 g, 8 mmol) were added to the reaction mass. After this, the reaction mass was refluxed for 1 h. Reaction completion was monitored using TLC, using a 1:1 (*v/v*) hexane:ethyl acetate mixture as an eluent.

After completion of the reaction, the solution was cooled to room temperature, then using a 10 % HCl solution, the pH was adjusted to 6.5–7. The solution was added dropwise to 50 mL of water under vigorous stirring. A white precipitate was formed. The precipitate was recrystallised from 10 mL of 96% ethanol.

280 mg of crystalline white compound was obtained, and the isolation yield was 45%, melting point: 229–231 °C; ^{1}H NMR (DMSO-*d6*, 500 MHz) δ (ppm): 11.98 (s, 1H, -NH), 7.22 (d, 2H, *J* = *8.8 Hz*, 2′-H, 6′-H), 7.16 (d, 2H, *J* = *8.8 Hz*, 2″-H, 6″-H), 6.97 (d, 2H, *J* = *8.8 Hz*, 3″-H, 5″-H), 6.88 (d, 2H, *J* = *8.8 Hz*, 3′-H, 5′-H), 4.03 (q, 2H, *J* = *6.9 Hz*, -O-CH_2), 3.72 (s, 3H, -O-CH_3), 1.33 (t, 3H, -CH_2CH_3); ^{13}C NMR (DMSO-*d6*, 125 MHz) δ (ppm): 160.6 (4′-C), 158.7 (4″-C), 155.3 (3-C), 145.8 (5-C), 129.6 (2″-C, 6″-C), 129.5 (2′-C, 6′-C), 126.7 (1″-C), 119.9 (1′-C), 115.3 (3″-C, 5″-C), 114.4 (3′-C, 5′-C), 63.8 (-O-CH_2), 55.6 (-O-CH_3), 15.0 (-CH_2-CH_3); ^{15}N NMR (DMSO-*d6*, 50 MHz) δ (ppm): 254.5 (1-N), 164.5 (2-N),

154.1 (4-N), FT-IR (cm^{-1}): 2974 ($\nu^{as}_{CH3\text{-}OR}$), 1698 ($\nu_{C=O}$), 1612 ($\nu_{sk.ar.}$), 1513 ($\nu_{sk.ar.}$), 1298 (ν^{as}_{COC}), 838 ($\gamma_{1,4\text{-disubst. phenyl}}$); HRMS-ESI (*m/z*): [M + Na^+] for $C_{17}H_{17}N_3O_3$ Na, calcd. 334.11621, found 334.11619.

All spectra are reported in supplementary materials.

5. Conclusions

A new triazolone **(3)** was synthesized by a new, unreported method, which probably followed a nucleophilic substitution of the alkylsulphanyl functional group with hydroxide anion. The reported method can potentially be used for the synthesis of similar triazolones.

Supplementary Materials: The following supporting information can be downloaded online. Figure S1. ^{1}H NMR spectrum of the compound **(2)**, Figure S2. ^{13}C NMR spectrum of the compound **(2)**, Figure S3. ^{13}C DEPT135 spectrum of the compound **(2)**, Figure S4. COSY ^{1}H-^{1}H spectrum of the compound **(2)**, Figure S5. HSQC ^{1}H-^{13}C spectrum of the compound **(2)**, Figure S6. HMBC ^{1}H-^{15}N spectrum of the compound **(2)**, Figure S7. HMBC ^{1}H-^{13}C spectrum of the compound **(2)**, Figure S8. ^{1}H NMR spectrum of the compound **(3)**, Figure S9. ^{13}C NMR spectrum of the compound **(3)**, Figure S10. ^{13}C DEPT135 spectrum of the compound **(3)**, Figure S11. COSY ^{1}H-^{1}H spectrum of the compound **(3)**, Figure S12. HSQC ^{1}H-^{13}C spectrum of the compound **(3)**, Figure S13. HSQC ^{1}H-^{15}N spectrum of the compound **(3)**, Figure S14. HMBC ^{1}H-^{13}C spectrum of the compound **(3)**, Figure S15. HMBC ^{1}H-^{15}N spectrum of the compound **(3)**, Figure S16. FT-IR spectrum of the compound **(2)**, Figure S17. FT-IR spectrum of the compound **(3)**, and Figure S18. HRMS spectrum of the compound **(3)**.

Author Contributions: Designed the experiments, V.B. and V.-N.B.; performed the experiments, I.B.; analysed the spectral data, V.B. and C.D.; wrote the manuscript, I.B.; supervision and funding acquisitions, V.B. and F.P. All authors have read and agreed to the published version of the manuscript.

Funding: This work was supported by a grant of the Ministry of Research, Innovation and Digitization, CNCS/CCCDI—UEFISCDI, project number PN-III-P2-2.1-PED-2019-3414, within PNCDI III.

Data Availability Statement: The data presented in this study are available within the article or supplementary material.

Conflicts of Interest: The authors declare that they have no conflict of interest.

References

1. Ferreira, V.F.; da Rocha, D.R.; da Silva, F.C.; Ferreira, P.G.; Boechat, N.A.; Magalhães, J.L. Novel 1*H*-1,2,3-, 2H-1,2,3-, 1*H*-1,2,4- and 4*H*-1,2,4-Triazole Derivatives: A Patent Review (2008–2011). *Expert Opin. Ther. Pat.* **2013**, *23*, 319–331. [CrossRef] [PubMed]
2. Küçükgüzel, Ş.G.; Çıkla-Süzgün, P. Recent Advances Bioactive 1,2,4-Triazole-3-Thiones. *Eur. J. Med. Chem.* **2015**, *97*, 830–870. [CrossRef] [PubMed]
3. Šermukšnytė, A.; Kantminienė, K.; Jonuškienė, I.; Tumosienė, I.; Petrikaitė, V. The Effect of 1,2,4-Triazole-3-Thiol Derivatives Bearing Hydrazone Moiety on Cancer Cell Migration and Growth of Melanoma, Breast, and Pancreatic Cancer Spheroids. *Pharmaceuticals* **2022**, *15*, 1026. [CrossRef] [PubMed]
4. Patel, K.R.; Brahmbhatt, J.G.; Pandya, P.A.; Daraji, D.G.; Patel, H.D.; Rawal, R.M.; Baran, S.K. Design, Synthesis and Biological Evaluation of Novel 5-(4-Chlorophenyl)-4-Phenyl-4H-1,2,4-Triazole-3-Thiols as an Anticancer Agent. *J. Mol. Struct.* **2021**, *1231*, 130000. [CrossRef]
5. El Ashry, E.S.H.; Farahat, M.M.K.; Awad, L.F.; Balbaa, M.; Yusef, H.; Badawy, M.E.I.; Abd Al Moaty, M.N. New 4-(Arylidene)Amino-1,2,4-Traizole-5-Thiol Derivatives and Their Acyclo Thioglycosides as α-Glucosidase and α-Amylase Inhibitors: Design, Synthesis, and Molecular Modelling Studies. *J. Mol. Struct.* **2022**, *1259*, 132733. [CrossRef]
6. Ihnatova, T.; Kaplaushenko, A.; Frolova, Y.; Pryhlo, E. Synthesis and Antioxidant Properties of Some New 5-Phenethyl-3-Thio-1,2,4-Triazoles. *Pharmacia* **2021**, *68*, 129–133. [CrossRef]
7. Domyati, D.; Zabin, S.A.; Elhenawy, A.A.; Abdelbaset, M. Preparation, Antimicrobial Activity and Docking Study of Vanadium Mixed Ligand Complexes Containing 4-Amino-5-Hydrazinyl-4*H*-1,2,4-Triazole-3-Thiol and Aminophenol Derivatives. *Processes* **2021**, *9*, 1008. [CrossRef]
8. Arustamyan, Z.S.; Margaryan, R.E.; Aghekyan, A.A.; Panosyan, G.A.; Muradyan, R.E.; Tumajyan, A.E. Synthesis and Anti-Inflammatory Properties of Substituted 5-(Tetrahydro-4-Phenyl-2*H*-Pyran-4-Yl)-4*H*-1,2,4-Triazole-3-Thiols. *Russ. J. Org. Chem.* **2021**, *57*, 195–202. [CrossRef]
9. Venugopala, K.N.; Kandeel, M.; Pillay, M.; Deb, P.K.; Abdallah, H.H.; Mahomoodally, M.F.; Chopra, D. Anti-Tubercular Properties of 4-Amino-5-(4-Fluoro-3- Phenoxyphenyl)-4*H*-1,2,4-Triazole-3-Thiol and Its Schiff Bases: Computational Input and Molecular Dynamics. *Antibiotics* **2020**, *9*, 559. [CrossRef]

10. Shah, S.A.A.; Ashraf, M.; Rehman, J.; Saleem, R.S.Z. Synthesis, in Vitro and in Silico Studies of S-Alkylated 5-(4-Methoxyphenyl)-4-Phenyl-4*H*-1,2,4-Triazole-3-Thiols as Cholinesterase Inhibitors. *Pak. J. Pharm. Sci.* **2018**, *31*, 2697–2708.
11. Ünver, Y.; Deniz, S.; Çelik, F.; Akar, Z.; Küçük, M.; Sancak, K. Synthesis of New 1,2,4-Triazole Compounds Containing Schiff and Mannich Bases (Morpholine) with Antioxidant and Antimicrobial Activities. *J. Enzym. Inhib. Med. Chem.* **2016**, *31* (Suppl. S3), 89–95. [CrossRef]
12. Tumosienė, I.; Jonuškienė, I.; Kantminienė, K.; Šiugždaitė, J.; Mickevičius, V.; Beresnevičius, Z.J. Synthesis and Biological Activity of 1,3,4-Oxa(Thia)Diazole, 1,2,4-Triazole-5-(Thio)One and S-Substituted Derivatives of 3-((2-Carboxyethyl)Phenylamino)Propanoic Acid. *Res. Chem. Intermed.* **2016**, *42*, 4459–4477. [CrossRef]
13. Ebrahimi, S.; Sayadi, M. Syntheses of Some Novel and Symmetrical Bis(4-Amino-4*H*-1,2,4-Triazole-3-Thiols). *J. Sulphur. Chem.* **2012**, *33*, 647–652. [CrossRef]
14. Altowyan, M.S.; Haukka, M.; Soliman, S.M.; Barakat, A.; Boraei, A.T.A.; Aboelmagd, A. Stereoselective Synthesis of New 4-Aryl-5-Indolyl-1,2,4-Triazole S- and N-β-Galactosides: Characterizations, X-Ray Crystal Structure and Hirshfeld Surface Analysis. *Crystals* **2023**, *13*, 797. [CrossRef]
15. Il'inykh, E.S.; Kim, D.G.; Valova, M.S.; Fedorova, O.V. Synthesis and Optical Properties of New S-Derivatives of 5,5′-(1,4-Phenylene)Bis(4H-1,2,4-Triazole-3-Thiol) and 5,5′,5″-(Benzene-1,3,5-Triyl)Tris(4H-1,2,4-Triazole-3-Thiol). *Russ. J. Gen. Chem.* **2019**, *89*, 2571–2576. [CrossRef]
16. Salvatore, R.N.; Smith, R.A.; Nischwitz, A.K.; Gavin, T. A Mild and Highly Convenient Chemoselective Alkylation of Thiols Using Cs_2CO_3–TBAI. *Tetrahedron Lett.* **2005**, *46*, 8931–8935. [CrossRef]
17. Socea, L.; Barbuceanu, S.; Socea, B.; Draghici, C.; Apostol, T.-V.; Pahontu, E.; Olaru, O. New Heterocyclic Compounds from 1,2,4-Triazoles Class with Potential Cytotoxic Activity. *Rev. Chim.* **2017**, *68*, 2503–2508. [CrossRef]
18. Deligeorgiev, T.; Kaloyanova, S.; Lesev, N.; Vaquero, J.J. An Easy and Fast Ultrasonic Selective S-Alkylation of Hetaryl Thiols at Room Temperature. *Ultrason. Sonochem.* **2010**, *17*, 783–788. [CrossRef]
19. Zheng, Y.; Wang, S.-B.; Cao, X.; Liu, D.-C.; Shu, B.; Quan, Z.-S. Design, Synthesis and Anticonvulsant Activity Evaluation of Novel 4-(4-Substitutedphenyl)-3-Methyl-1*H*-1,2,4-Triazol-5(4*H*)-Ones. *Drug Res.* **2013**, *64*, 40–46. [CrossRef]
20. An, F.; Xuan, X.; Liu, Z.; Bian, M.; Shen, Q.; Quan, Z.; Zhang, G.; Wei, C. Anti-Inflammatory Activity of 4-(4-(Heptyloxy)Phenyl)-2,4-Dihydro-3H-1,2,4-Triazol-3-One via Repression of MAPK/NF-KB Signaling Pathways in β-Amyloid-Induced Alzheimer's Disease Models. *Molecules* **2022**, *27*, 5035. [CrossRef]
21. Ustabaş, R.; Süleymanoğlu, N.; Ünver, Y.; Direkel, Ş. 5-(4-Bromobenzyl)-4-(4-(5-Phenyl-1,3,4-Oxadiazole-2-Yl)Phenyl)-2,4-Dihydro-3H-1,2,4-Triazole-3-One: Synthesis, Characterization, DFT Study and Antimicrobial Activity. *J. Mol. Struct.* **2020**, *1214*, 128217. [CrossRef]
22. Malbec, F.; Milcent, R.; Vicart, P.; Bure, A.M. Synthesis of New Derivatives of 4-Amino-2,4-Dihydro-1,2,4-Triazol-3-One as Potential Antibacterial Agents. *J. Heterocycl. Chem.* **1984**, *21*, 1769–1774. [CrossRef]
23. Sirach, R.R.; Dave, P.N. 3-Nitro-1,2,4-Triazol-5-One (NTO): High Explosive Insensitive Energetic Material. *Chem. Heterocycl. Comp.* **2021**, *57*, 720–730. [CrossRef]
24. Kikugawa, Y.; Yamada, S.; Nagashima, H.; Kaji, K. The Reaction of Substituted Ureas with Sodium Borohydride in Pyridine. *Tetrahedron. Lett.* **1969**, *10*, 699–702. [CrossRef]
25. Molla, E.; Abser, N.; Islam, M. Synthesis and Characterization of Some 4-Aryl Substituted Thiosemicarbazides, N-Alkyloxybenzaldehydes Containing Long Alkyl Chains and Their Corresponding Thiosemicarbazones. *Jahangirnagar. Univ. J. Sci.* **2018**, *41*, 31–42.
26. Siwek, A.; Wujec, M.; Dobosz, M.; Wawrzycka-Gorczyca, I. Study of Direction of Cyclization of 1-Azolil-4-Aryl/Alkyl-Thiosemicarbazides. *Heteroat. Chem.* **2010**, *21*, 521–532. [CrossRef]
27. Pareek, A.K.; Joseph, P.E.; Seth, D.S. Convenient Synthesis, Characterization of Some Novel Substituted 3-Methyl-2-Pyrazoline-5-Ones and Substituted 3,5-Dimethyl Pyrazoles. *Orient. J. Chem.* **2010**, *26*, 1467–1471.

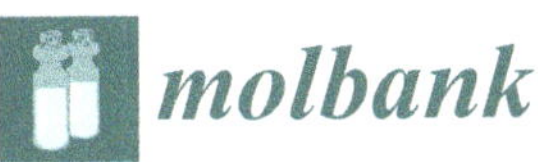 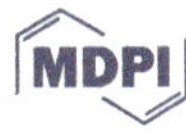

Short Note

2,8-Dibromo-6*H*,12*H*-6,12-epoxydibenzo[*b*,*f*][1,5]dioxocine

R. Alan Aitken *, David B. Cordes, An Jie Ler and Aidan P. McKay

EaStCHEM School of Chemistry, University of St Andrews, North Haugh, St Andrews KY16 9ST, Fife, UK
* Correspondence: raa@st-and.ac.uk; Tel.: +44-1334-463865

Abstract: The title dibromodisalicylaldehyde, obtained as a by-product in the *m*-chloroperoxybenzoic acid oxidation of 5-bromo-2-(methoxymethoxy)benzaldehyde, has been characterised by IR and NMR spectroscopy and X-ray diffraction. The structure features two independent molecules with a π–π stacking interaction between them.

Keywords: X-ray structure; disalicylaldehyde; trioxabicyclo[3.3.1]nonadiene

1. Introduction

Ever since salicylaldehyde **1** was first studied in the mid-19th century, it was observed to undergo dehydrative dimerisation, particularly under acidic conditions, to give a compound variously described as "parasalicyl" [1,2] and disalicylaldehyde [3]. There were various suggestions as to its structure and in a definitive paper of 1922 [4] this was finally shown by chemical methods to be the interesting dibenzo-fused trioxabicyclo[3.3.1]nonadiene **2** (Scheme 1). The activity of substituted derivatives of **2** as antimicrobial agents has been reported [5].

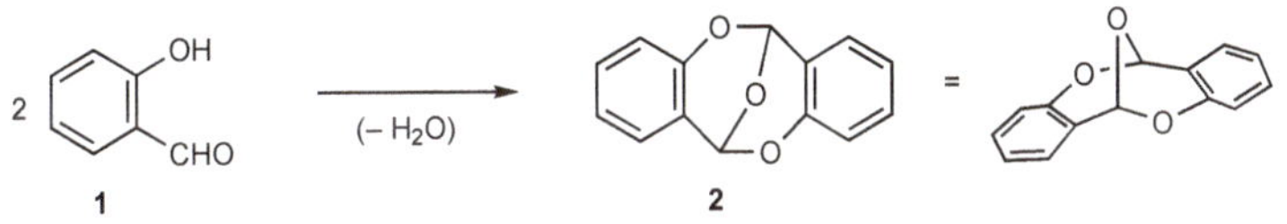

Scheme 1. Formation and structure of "disalicylaldehyde" **2**.

Citation: Aitken, R.A.; Cordes, D.B.; Ler, A.J.; McKay, A.P. 2,8-Dibromo-6*H*,12*H*-6,12-epoxydibenzo[*b*,*f*][1,5]dioxocine. *Molbank* **2023**, *2023*, M1729. https://doi.org/10.3390/M1729

Academic Editors: Stefano D'Errico and Annalisa Guaragna

Received: 24 August 2023
Revised: 16 September 2023
Accepted: 17 September 2023
Published: 19 September 2023

In the course of recent synthetic work, we were carrying out a Baeyer–Villiger oxidation of the methoxymethyl-ether-protected 5-bromosalicylaldehyde **3** to give the protected bromocatechol **4** and, in addition to the expected product, obtained a minor by-product in low yield which turned out to be the dibromo derivative of disalicylaldehyde **5** (Scheme 2). This has only been mentioned once before in a 1940 paper where it was obtained by direct bromination of **2** and only a melting point was given [6]. We describe here the full characterisation of this compound including its IR and NMR spectra and X-ray structure determination.

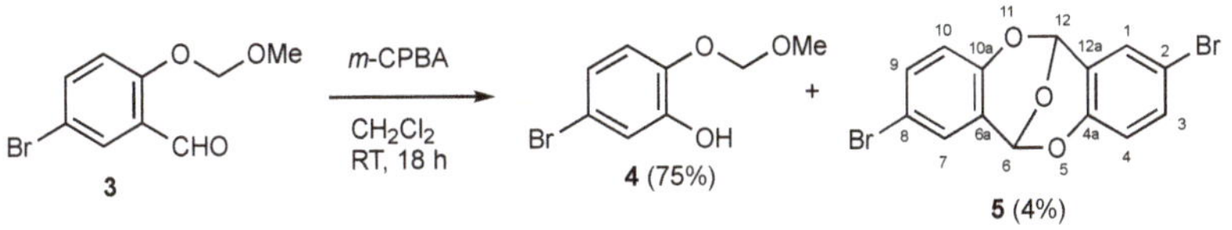

Scheme 2. Formation of compound **5**.

2. Results

The starting compound **3** was prepared according to a literature procedure [7] and subjected to *m*-chloroperoxybenzoic acid (*m*-CPBA) oxidation as described in a patent [8]. We faced significant difficulty in separating the desired product **4** from the *m*-chlorobenzoic acid and even after several washings had to subject the residue to column chromatography. This did give the required product **4** in 75% isolated yield after a further recrystallisation, but a fast-running minor component was also obtained which proved to be the unexpected dibromodisalicylaldehyde **5** (4%). In addition to NMR signals for a 1,2,4-trisubstituted benzene ring (see Supplementary Materials), this had a distinctive singlet at δ_H 6.28 and δ_C 89.4 ppm in agreement with expectation for a benzylic ArCH(OR)$_2$ environment. The IR spectrum showed no significant signals above 1650 cm^{-1} confirming the absence of OH and C=O. The material failed to give any meaningful mass spectrometric data.

Recrystallisation from hexane gave colourless prisms suitable for X-ray diffraction and the resulting structure (Figure 1) shows two independent but closely similar molecules in the unit cell. At 1.888(8)–1.892(8) Å the C–Br distances are rather short compared to the mean value of 1.899 Å for ArC–Br [9]. Two views of the molecule (Figure 2) show that the central trioxabicyclo[3.3.1] ring system is symmetrical and distinctly angular.

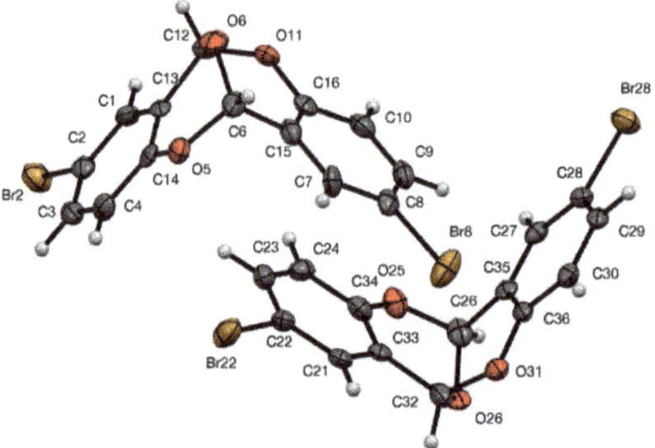

Figure 1. Molecular structure of **5** showing the two independent molecules with anisotropic displacement ellipsoids drawn at 50% probability level (hydrogen atoms are shown as grey spheres of arbitrary size) and the numbering system used.

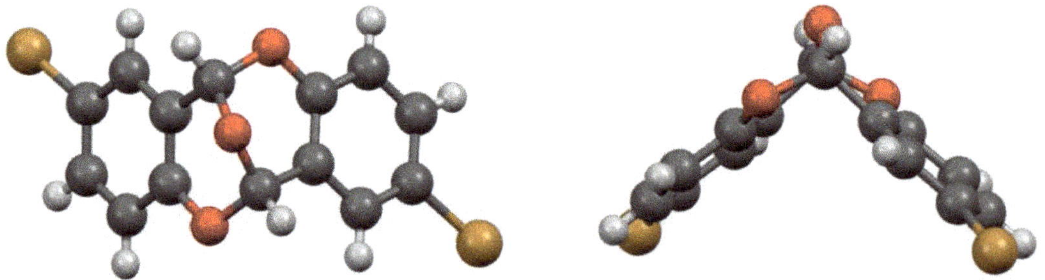

Figure 2. Two alternative views of **5** showing the symmetrical and distinctly angular shape of the molecule (carbon atoms—dark grey, hydrogen atoms—light grey, oxygen atoms—red, bromine atoms—brown).

As far as we are aware, only six compounds with this core structure have been previously characterised by X-ray diffraction (Figure 3) and the key geometric parameters for these are compared with **5** in Table 1. It can be seen that these form a relatively consistent pattern with the possible exception of the parent compound **2** which has longer bridging C–O bonds, a larger angle at the ring oxygens and a smaller angle between the mean planes. This last parameter is the angle between the planes defined by the five atoms making up each of the three-atom bridges in the bicyclo[3.3.1] system, i.e., CH–O–C=C–CH.

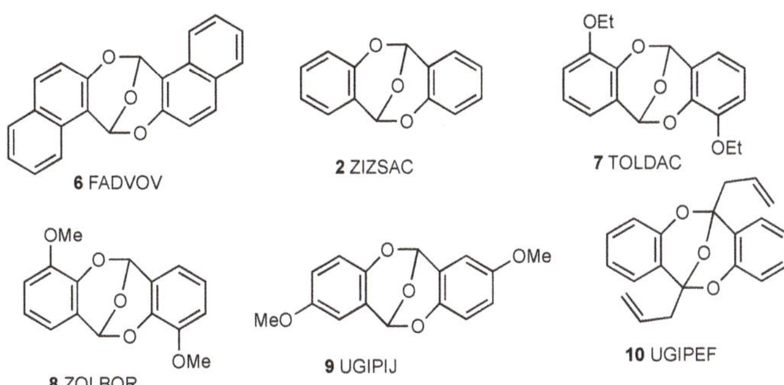

Figure 3. Crystallographically characterised disalicylaldehyde derivatives with CSD Ref Codes.

Table 1. Comparison of selected geometric parameters for **5** and related compounds (Å, °).

Compd	Bridging C–O Length (s)	Angle at Bridging O	Angle(s) at Ring Os	Angle between Mean Planes	Ref
5	1.404 (10), 1.410 (11)	109.6 (6)	111.6 (6), 112.4 (7)	72.9	This work
5	1.403 (11), 1.407 (11)	109.9 (6)	112.5 (6), 112.7 (6)	73.5	This work
6 FADVOV	1.418	108.6	112.3 (2)	71.7	[10]
2 ZIZSAC	1.549	106.5	117.9 (9)	65.9	[11]
7 TOLDAC	1.415(2), 1.417(2)	108.0(1)	111.4(1), 111.9(1)	73.5	[12]
8 ZOLBOR	1.411(3), 1.416(3)	107.8(2)	111.5(2), 111.7(2)	72.75	[13]
9 UGIPIJ	1.408(5), 1.414(5)	109.3(3)	112.2(2), 112.3(3)	72.75	[14]
10 UGIPEF	1.413(2), 1.417(2)	111.0(1)	112.6(1), 113.1(1)	73.6	[14]

The other main feature of the crystal structure of **5**, which is not evident in Figure 1, is the arrangement of adjacent pairs of independent molecules to allow a favourable π–π stacking interaction between them (Figure 4, distance between two mean planes 3.384 Å, centroid···centroid distance 3.602(6) Å). Among the six other structures of Figure 3 this feature only seems to occur for **2** (distance between two mean planes 3.264 Å). We assume that the presence of bulky substituents in the other cases prevents this arrangement.

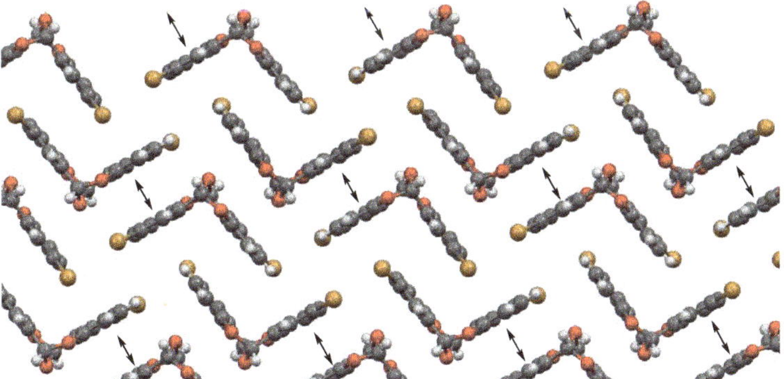

Figure 4. Crystal structure of **5** viewed along the crystallographic *a* axis showing π–π stacking interactions (arrows) between pairs of independent molecules.

In summary, the dibromodisalicylaldehyde **5** obtained as a minor by-product has been spectroscopically characterised for the first time and its X-ray crystal structure consist of pairs of independent molecules in a π–π stacking arrangement.

3. Experimental

Melting points were recorded on a Reichert hot-stage microscope (Reichert, Vienna, Austria) and are uncorrected. IR spectra were recorded using the ATR technique on a Shimadzu IRAffinity 1S instrument. NMR spectra were obtained using a Bruker AV300 instrument (Bruker, Billerica, MA, USA). Spectra were run with internal Me_4Si as the reference and chemical shifts are reported in ppm to high frequency of the reference.

3.1. *Reaction Leading to Formation of* 5

A solution of 5-bromo-2-methoxymethoxybenzaldehyde **3** [7] (20.0 g, 81.6 mmol) and *m*-chloroperoxybenzoic acid (28.8 g, 116.7 mmol) in CH_2Cl_2 (300 mL) was stirred at RT for 18 h. The mixture was filtered and the filtrate was stirred with 2 M aqueous $Na_2S_2O_3$ for 2 h. The organic layer was separated, dried and evaporated to give a solid (25.3 g). Column chromatography of this (SiO_2, hexane/EtOAc, 4:1) gave, as the first fraction, by-product **5** (0.66 g, 4%) followed by the desired product **4** (14.35 g, 75%) which had data in agreement with the published values [8].

Data for **5**: mp 157–159 °C (lit. [6] 168 °C); IR: ν_{max}/cm^{-1} 1607, 1477, 1412, 1265, 1221, 1184, 1132, 957, 881, 858, 814; ^1H NMR (300 MHz, $CDCl_3$, 25 °C): δ 6.28 (2H, s, OCHO, H-6,12), 6.79 (2H, d, *J* 6.6 Hz, H-4,10), 7.36 (2H, dd, *J* 6.6, 1.8 Hz, H-3,9), 7.42 (2H, d, *J* 1.8 Hz, H-1,7); ^{13}C NMR (75 MHz, $CDCl_3$, 25 °C): δ 89.4 (2CH, OCHO, C-6,12), 113.9 (2C, C-2,8), 118.6 (2CH, C-4,10), 121.3 (2C, C-6a,12a), 130.1 (2CH, C-1,7), 134.2 (2CH, C-3,9), 149.4 (2C, C-4a,10a). ^{13}C NMR assignments for CH confirmed by HSQC. Recrystallisation of **5** from hexane gave crystals suitable for X-ray diffraction.

3.2. *X-ray Structure Determination of* 5

X-ray diffraction data for compound **5** was collected at 173 K using a Rigaku FR-X Ultrahigh Brilliance Microfocus RA generator/confocal optics with XtaLAB P200 diffractometer [Mo Kα radiation (λ = 0.71073 Å)]. Data were collected and processed (including correction for Lorentz, polarization and absorption) using CrysAlisPro [15]. Structures were solved by dual-space methods (SHELXT) [16] and refined by full-matrix least-squares against F^2 (SHELXL-2019/3) [17]. Non-hydrogen atoms were refined anisotropically, and hydrogen atoms were refined using a riding model. All calculations were performed using the Olex2 [18] interface.

Crystal data for $C_{14}H_8Br_2O_3$, M = 384.02 g mol^{-1}, colourless prism, crystal dimensions 0.09 × 0.08 × 0.06 mm, triclinic, space group P-1 (No. 2), a = 6.9692(3), b = 9.2930(4), c = 21.4788(10) Å, α = 97.000(4), β = 97.013(4), γ = 110.805(4) °, V = 1270.00(10) $Å^3$, Z = 4, D_{calc} = 2.008 g cm^{-3}, T = 173 K, R_1 = 0.0798, wR_2 = 0.1442 for 4246 reflections with $I > 2\sigma(I)$ and 343 variables, R_{int} 0.0422, Goodness of fit on F^2 1.323. Data have been deposited at the Cambridge Crystallographic Data Centre as CCDC 2290326. The data can be obtained free of charge from the Cambridge Crystallographic Data Centre via http://www.ccdc.cam.ac.uk/getstructures.

Supplementary Materials: The following supporting information can be downloaded at: ^1H and ^{13}C and HSQC NMR and IR data as well as cif and check-cif files for **5**.

Author Contributions: A.J.L. prepared the compound, D.B.C. and A.P.M. collected the X-ray data and solved the structure; R.A.A. designed the study, analysed the data, and wrote the paper. All authors have read and agreed to the published version of the manuscript.

Funding: This research received no external funding.

Data Availability Statement: The X-ray data are at CCDC as stated in the paper.

Conflicts of Interest: The authors declare no conflict of interest.

References

1. Ettling. Ueber die Distillationsproducte des salicyligsauren und benzoësauren Kupferoxyds. *Liebigs Ann. Chem.* **1845**, *53*, 77–90. [CrossRef]
2. Cahours, A. Untersuchungen über das Phenol (Phenylhydrat). *Liebigs Ann. Chem.* **1851**, *78*, 225–228. [CrossRef]
3. Perkin, W.H. Ueber Benzosalicyl- und Disalicylwasserstoff. *Liebigs Ann. Chem.* **1868**, *145*, 295–301. [CrossRef]
4. Adams, R.; Fogler, M.F.; Kreger, C.W. The structure of disalicyl aldehyde. *J. Am. Chem. Soc.* **1922**, *44*, 1126–1133. [CrossRef]
5. Fiedler, H. Derivate des 2-Hydroxy-3-methoxy-benzaldehyds. *Arch. Pharm.* **1964**, *297*, 226–235. [CrossRef] [PubMed]
6. Tamaki, T.; Endo, Z. Action of phosphorus pentoxide on organic compounds I. Reaction between salicylaldehyde and phosphorus pentoxide. *Nippon Kagaku Kaishi* **1940**, *61*, 231–233.
7. Nevesely, T.; Daniliuc, C.G.; Gilmour, R. Sequential energy transfer catalysis: A cascade synthesis of angularly-fused dihydrocoumarins. *Org. Lett.* **2019**, *21*, 9724–9728. [CrossRef] [PubMed]
8. Hagihara, M.; Tanaka, M.; Katsube, T.; Okudo, M.; Iwase, N.; Shigetomi, M.; Kanda, T.; Nakanishi, T. Pyrrolopyridazinone Compound. European Patent 1982986 A1, 22 October 2008.
9. Allen, F.H.; Kennard, O.; Watson, D.G.; Brammer, L.; Orpen, A.G.; Taylor, R. Tables of bond lengths determined by X-ray and neutron diffraction. Part 1. Bond lengths in organic compounds. *J. Chem. Soc. Perkin Trans. 2* **1987**, S1–S19. [CrossRef]
10. Bachet, B.; Brassy, C.; Guidi-Morosini, C. Epoxy-8,16 Dihydro-8,16 Dinaphto[2,1-*b*:2′,1′-*f*][dioxocinne-1,5]. *Acta Crystallogr. Sect. C* **1986**, *42*, 1630–1632. [CrossRef]
11. Vol'eva, V.B.; Belostotskaya, I.S.; Shishkin, O.V.; Struchkov, Y.T.; Ershov, V.V. Synthesis and structures of anhydrodimers of salicylaldehydes. *Russ. Chem. Bull.* **1995**, *44*, 1489–1491. [CrossRef]
12. Wang, L.-H.; Lin, D.-D. The crystal structure of 4,10-ethoxy-6*H*,12*H*-6,12-epoxydibenzo[*b*,*f*][1,5]dioxocine, $C_{18}H_{18}O_5$. *Z. Kristallogr. New Cryst. Struct.* **2019**, *234*, 673–674. [CrossRef]
13. Stomberg, R.; Li, S.; Lindquist, K. Crystal structure of 4,10-dimethoxy-6,12-epoxy-6*H*,12*H*-dibenzo[*b*,*f*][1,5]dioxocin, $C_{16}H_{14}O_5$. *Z. Kristallogr. Cryst. Mater.* **1995**, *210*, 967–968. [CrossRef]
14. Ragot, J.P.; Prime, M.E.; Archibald, S.J.; Taylor, R.J.K. A novel route to preussomerins via 2-arylacetal anions. *Org. Lett.* **2000**, *2*, 1613–1616. [CrossRef] [PubMed]
15. *CrysAlisPro*, v1.171.42.94a; Rigaku Oxford Diffraction, Rigaku Corporation: Tokyo, Japan, 2023.
16. Sheldrick, G.M. SHELXT—Integrated space-group and crystal structure determination. *Acta Crystallogr. Sect. A Found. Adv.* **2015**, *71*, 3–8. [CrossRef] [PubMed]
17. Sheldrick, G.M. Crystal structure refinement with SHELXL. *Acta Crystallogr. Sect. C Struct. Chem.* **2015**, *71*, 3–8. [CrossRef] [PubMed]
18. Dolomanov, O.V.; Bourhis, L.J.; Gildea, R.J.; Howard, J.A.K.; Puschmann, H. OLEX2: A complete structure solution, refinement and analysis program. *J. Appl. Crystallogr.* **2009**, *42*, 339–341. [CrossRef]

MDPI
St. Alban-Anlage 66
4052 Basel
Switzerland
www.mdpi.com

Molbank Editorial Office
E-mail: molbank@mdpi.com
www.mdpi.com/journal/molbank

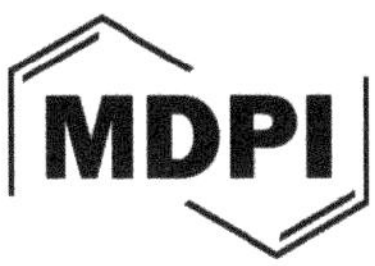

www.ingramcontent.com/pod-product-compliance
Lightning Source LLC
LaVergne TN
LVHW070643170726
843515LV00004B/311

* 9 7 8 3 0 3 6 5 9 2 8 2 4 *